Transitions
Managing Your Own Healthcare
What Every Teen with an LSD Needs to Know

Written by
Dawn A. Laney, MS, CGC,
Carol Ogg, BS Pharm,
and Nadia Ali, PhD

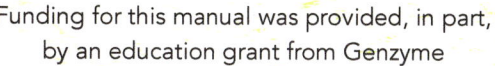

Funding for this manual was provided, in part,
by an education grant from Genzyme

DEDICATION

To Dr. Paul Fernhoff who always encouraged us to bring our ideas to fruition, and to all the individuals who have let us join them on their journey to becoming amazing adults.

Proceeds from the sale of this workbook will be donated to the Paul M. Fernhoff endowment fund

Table of Contents

Chapter One
What every teen needs to know to manage their healthcare

So, What is a Transition?

A transition is a move from one place or stage of life to another. Being in transition means being in-between, going through changes—and as with any changes, there are new things to learn. In your case, one of the many transitions you're making as a teen is learning how to manage your own health rather than having your parents do it for you. That can be very exciting and a little scary all at the same time. The good news is you are not alone during this transition. Your family, friends, healthcare team, and this workbook are here to help you figure things out! Feel free to read this book straight through or jump to the exercises or topics that apply most to you.

A Focus on Teens (i.e. YOU!)

The teenage years are the time when teens often begin separating their thoughts, goals, and self-image from those of their parents. Teens begin exploring who they are and who they want to become as they enter adulthood. For people living with a chronic condition, like a lysosomal storage disease, the teen years should also include a gradual transfer of medical care responsibility from parents to the teens themselves. As you might guess, it's a lot easier to learn to do this slowly and with a plan, rather than jumping headfirst into a fast and confusing crash course of medical needs on your 18th birthday. So, let's start making a plan!

The goal of *Transitions: Managing Your Own Healthcare* is exactly what the title says; it is a learning workbook to help prepare you to successfully manage your own healthcare. To be successful, this means involving not only you and your parents, but also other family members, healthcare professionals and related community agencies. We want to help you build a plan that recognizes your current strengths, interests, and preferences, while also figuring out what services and support you need to reach your goal of successfully managing your own healthcare. We'll explore each of these items at length in this workbook.

Well, Everyone Does It!

First of all, it's important to remember that all of us go through transitions as we get older and make the change from a child into an adult: we move from pediatrics into adult medicine, leave high school to begin a job or enter college, and move from our parents' insurance to our own insurance. We may also move out of our parents' home into our own home, learn to pay bills and/or maybe even get married. Your doctors had to do it. Your parents had to do it. You have to do it. Although we eagerly look forward to some of these changes, it often doesn't occur to us to begin learning how to take ownership of our health. Yet our health influences all aspects of our lives. *So, for each and every one of us, transition includes preparing to manage our own healthcare.*

For you, as a teen living with a lysosomal storage disease, the medical part of the transition can be a little more complicated. We want to help you make the move as smoothly as possible—from other people managing your healthcare to *you managing your healthcare*. As you become a young adult, learning how to take responsibility for your own healthcare can be a rich and rewarding experience. Assuming responsibility for your own healthcare is the ultimate goal of this learning workbook.

This workbook, *Transitions: Managing Your Own Healthcare*, is packed full of exercises designed to help you figure out how much you already are managing your own healthcare and how to uncover what you still need to learn and master. Remember, the process starts around 14 years of age, so some exercises may seem simple to you if you are 21 years old. Even so, we highly recommend that you do all the exercises, as there are a lot of things you can learn from each section.

Chapter Two

"The Top 10 Tips"

*We recommend these "Top 10 Tips" for preparing
to manage your own healthcare:*

1. **Start early!** The early teen years are a great time to communicate and plan. Begin with a meeting to put together a transition plan. This meeting should include you, your parents and the members of your core medical team. It should include a discussion about the importance of self-directed medical care as you enter adulthood. If you can start by talking with your parents and healthcare providers, it can make the transition easier and give you the chance to learn more about how to do it.

2. **Take a quick test.** Before starting off on your transition journey, figuring out what you already know is as important as figuring out what you don't know. What do you know about your disease, your treatment, and your overall medical care? Basic healthcare questionnaires, like the "Ready to Manage Your Own Health Care?," created by the PACER Center, Inc. and modified for teens with lysosomal storage diseases, are a great start and can direct you to areas that need attention. We've included a specialized version of the form in the back of this workbook in Chapter 5.

3. **Know your disease and treatment plan.** Teens should work closely with their healthcare providers to understand their disease and what needs to be done to keep them as healthy as possible. It is important for you to learn why you do all that you do medically (treatments, pills, doctor's appointments, and tests). If you understand how and why you do things, it helps you know how to rank them in importance in day-to-day life. It can also be helpful to create a disease and treatment summary sheet. We have examples of these forms and applications in Chapter 9.

4. **Know your healthcare providers.** It is important for you to know each of your doctors/healthcare providers and what they do. Make a list with contact information for each of your doctors/healthcare providers and their medical specialties, so you'll have it when you need it. This knowledge will help you know how and when to contact the correct healthcare provider during a medical issue. See a sample list in Chapter 9.

5. Learn about insurance. It is important for you to understand and discuss insurance with your health providers, parents and/or case managers. Important points to talk about may include: 1) why insurance is needed and 2) how insurance availability changes over time. It is also critical that you know what happens to your insurance in different life scenarios, like dropping out of school, turning 26 years of age or going to a vocational school.

6. Plan for adulthood. You may be asked to think about what you'd like to do over the next few years and discuss it with your parents and healthcare providers. Do you want to continue in school after high school? Do you want to work right away? Do you want to volunteer? What would be a realistic dream job? Your parents and healthcare providers can work together with you to help you understand how to make your goals a reality, and discuss practical issues, like your insurance, that often go hand in hand.

7. Meet your new doctors. Some providers, like many medical geneticists and/or genetic counselors, are able to work with patients for their entire life. Other doctors, like pediatricians, may only extend their services until you turn 18 or 21 years of age. A change from "kid-focused doctors" to "adult doctors" can be easier if you and your parents know who your new doctors are and meet them before it is officially time to begin working with them.

8. Learn when a health issue requires treatment. As you know, some health issues are more serious than others. Your healthcare providers and parents can help you learn when a stomach ache is something that your doctor needs to know about immediately, or something which can be treated with an over-the-counter medication from the drugstore and/or waiting for it to go away.

9. Advocate for yourself and know your resources. You know yourself best, so you must become involved in your healthcare. You need to teach other people about your disease and needs. You need to know where to turn for information. You are your best advocate and your best resource! You also need to know that it is OK to speak up if you are uncomfortable with a healthcare provider or if you need a little more explanation about something before doing it. **Remember, you are in charge of your healthcare.**

10. DON'T PANIC! It may seem like a lot right now – so many things to do and know! - but millions of teens move from being a kid to an adult every year. With a little planning and participation from everyone, this can be a smooth transition.

Chapter Three

Your Biggest Concerns

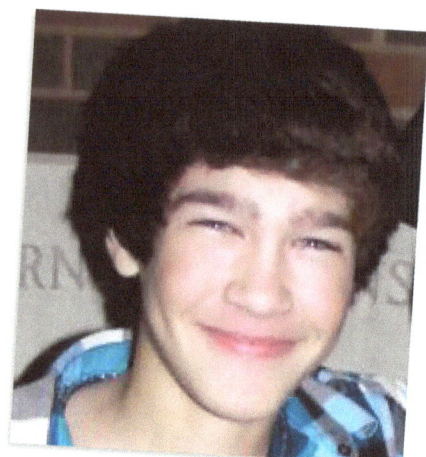

For many teens, transitioning from their teenage years to adulthood is a major milestone. Great pride and joy comes to some teens as they move out of their parents' house and into their college dorm. For others, they can't wait to get their first job, start a vocational school, or take on new responsibilities. Almost every teen will experience more independence than they did at a younger age. Along with all these exciting events can come worries. This next exercise will help you identify your concerns, worries, fears or issues so you can face them, work with them, and find the necessary skills to master them.

Brian, a tall, dark-haired 24-year-old was diagnosed with Fabry disease as a teenager after years of looking for a reason for his horrible stomach aches and frequent burning pain in his hands and feet. Thinking back, he remembers:

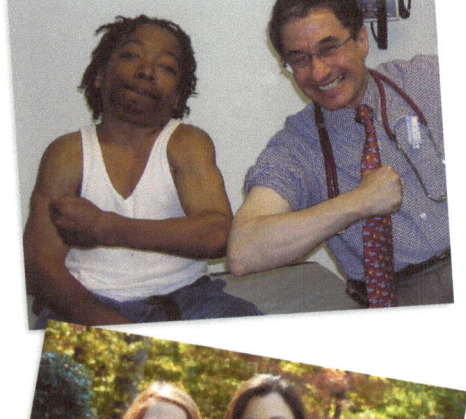

> "I first understood that I had Fabry disease when I was 14 or 15 years old and at that point all the decisions about my medical care were made by my mom or the doctors. By the time I was 18 or 19 years old I began making my own treatment decisions. It is important to me to make sure to stay informed about what is new in research for my condition and feel OK talking to the doctors, nurses, and genetic counselors about it."
>
> Brian, a 24-year-old with Fabry disease

We've surveyed other teens living with a lysosomal storage disease and have listed the *Top 10 Concerns* they shared as they transitioned from being a teenager to managing their own healthcare as an adult. You might share some of the same concerns listed on the next page, or your concerns, fears and anxieties may be quite different. These Top 10 Concerns are not listed in any particular order.

Top 10 Concerns

Exercise: Read through the concerns below and place a check mark next to each one if you can relate to it. We have included space at the end of this section to record any additional concerns if they are not listed here.

- [ ] **1.** My parent(s) just won't let go and let me make the transition on my own.

- [ ] **2.** I'm worried that I won't know the difference between an emergency (go to the ER) and a minor illness (call your doctor and/or go to urgent care).

- [ ] **3.** I'm worried about managing my treatments by myself.

- [ ] **4.** I'm worried that my nurse will do things differently than I'm used to and I won't know how to talk to her/him.

- [ ] **5.** I am worried about making my own doctor's appointments and transitioning to adult medicine.

- [ ] **6.** I'm worried about insurance coverage and doctors' bills.

- [ ] **7.** I'm worried about getting transportation to my appointments and infusions.

- [ ] **8.** I'm concerned that when I can make my own medical decisions I won't want to do my infusions anymore.

- [ ] **9.** I'm worried that I don't understand my disease or treatments well enough to make good decisions and get the best medical care.

- [ ] **10.** I don't want anyone to know that I have a lysosomal storage disease.

Your Biggest Concerns Exercise

*Like most teens, you probably made more than three check marks in the previous exercise. That's OK. For this exercise, though, rank your **Top 3 Concerns** and transfer them to the blank spaces below. If you have a concern that is not listed and you rank it amongst your Top 3, use the space provided below to write it down.*

1. _____

   _____

   _____

2. _____

   _____

   _____

3. _____

   _____

   _____

Now that we've identified your Top 3 Concerns, you will want to keep this page handy and refer back to it. *Tip: Use a sticky note, bookmark or a doctor's business card to mark your place so it is easy to find it again.*

Each of your Top 10 Concerns is important and real. The goal is to give you the necessary tools to help find answers to these valid concerns. In adulthood, solving your own problems, or getting the right help to solve your problems, is very important for your own growth and development.

Let's Talk More About Your Concerns

1. My parent/guardian just won't let go and let me do this on my own.

"Even though I thought I could totally be responsible for making my own appointments, my parents figured it'd be like the hamster I had when I was 10 and I'd mess it up. They were sure that I'd forget something important and then I would be back to feeling bad again. They kept checking up on me and it got really annoying."

Mary, a 20-year-old with MPSI, remembers her top concern from the past

For many years, your parent(s) have made all the decisions for you about medical insurance, physicians, treatments, etc. Many parents have commented that the reason they were so afraid to turn everything over to their teen is that managing your healthcare is complicated and they would hate to see the same mistakes made twice. Growing up is hard for teens, but it is sometimes harder for the parents to recognize that their teen is indeed ready to assume responsibility.

The earlier you start the process of managing your own healthcare, the easier it will be to take full responsibility. Think of it this way: you have to get your learner's permit prior to getting your actual driver's license. And why is that? You need experience! You first learn to drive in an open parking lot long before you attempt the interstate at 65 miles an hour. You have to prove to your parents that you really can be trusted and you understand the rules of the road.

The same is true of managing your own healthcare. You can't just leave the house at 18 years of age and say you're ready if you don't even understand the fundamentals of your disease. So what can you do? At age 14, you can become involved in understanding your disease and treatment. Ask questions of your parents, nurse, and physician. Show that you are taking an active role.

This basic understanding of your lysosomal storage disease can be as simple as the following:

"My lysosomal storage disease is caused because I am missing an enzyme (or have a reduced amount of a certain enzyme). As a result, my body is not able to break down a specific substance (a lipid) and it stores it in various places in my body.

Just like kids with diabetes have to take insulin to replace what they don't have, I have to take pills every day to reduce the stuff (lipids) stored in my cells or get regular infusions to replace the missing enzyme.

It's really important that I take my medication or get my infusions on a regular schedule because once the lipid builds up to a certain point and causes irreversible damage, it's hard for any amount of enzyme to fix the problem."

Sometimes when your parents have always done things for you, you may be tempted to continue on this path and let them continue to "always do it for you." However, come 18 years of age when you are facing the inevitable, you'll find that pre-planning definitely will pay off. At age 16, with your parent(s) at your side, ask if you can make your next annual appointment with your primary physician. At this stage, you should write that phone number down or enter it into your contacts list.

Exercise: At your next appointment with your primary care physician and/or geneticist, pay close attention to who answers the questions the doctor asks. This is a good sign of who is managing your disease. If your parents answer all the questions and you don't have much chance to answer, now is the time to discuss this with your parents. Before your next scheduled visit, it is important to talk to your parents about your taking an active role in answering the questions yourself! They can always add anything you forget after you've finished answering.

There is an old saying: "You have to walk before you run." Remember, your parents are going through this transition too! It may be difficult for them to see you as independent and grown up. This will take time for everyone, one step at a time. The earlier you start this transition, the easier it will be for everyone.

2. I'm worried that I won't know the difference between an emergency (go to the hospital emergency room) and an illness (call your doctor).

"OK, so seriously...how do I know if the pain in my chest is just from carrying my overloaded messenger bag or is a heart attack?"

Troy, a 16-year-old living with Gaucher disease

This is a common concern, expressed by many teens as a major fear entering adulthood. When is a headache just a headache or when does it need immediate attention? When in doubt, always trust your instincts and call your doctor. They will either tell you what to do at home, have you come into their office for an evaluation or direct you to rush to the nearest emergency room.

For children and teens, a few of the signs that should be brought to the attention of a healthcare professional immediately include:[1]

- A bluish tint to the skin, fingernails, lips, tongue and/or other parts of the body. The blue color is a sign indicating a lack of oxygen.
- Difficulty breathing
- Sluggishness, extreme tiredness
- Trembling or seizures
- High fever

It is not uncommon for a teen to experience chest pain. Believe it or not, this can be perfectly harmless and be caused by growing pains. However, only a doctor can determine the cause of chest pains. If you have chest pain, pressure or chest discomfort, call your doctor immediately.

It is also advisable to call your doctor if you experience any unexpected problems in thinking or you find yourself feeling or acting strangely, as this may indicate a stroke or other serious medical issue. Although strokes are not very common in children and young adults, always err on the side of caution and call your doctor immediately with symptoms of numbness, especially on one side of the body, slurred speech, or a debilitating (i.e. really, really, really bad!) headache.

Don't forget about your mental health too! We have focused on answering questions with a focus on physical symptoms, but transitions are a time of mental stress too. We know that some patients living with LSDs may have depression, panic attacks, and increased anxiety as part of their disease's symptoms. If you find that you are having any symptoms such as those listed below please contact your health care team.

- Difficulty concentrating, remembering details, and making decisions
- Fatigue and decreased energy
- Feelings of guilt, worthlessness, and/or helplessness
- Feeling irritable, restless or agitated
- Feelings of hopelessness and/or pessimism
- Feeling very tense or uneasy in situations that would not have bothered you much in the past.
- Insomnia, early-morning wakefulness, or excessive sleeping
- Loss of interest in activities or hobbies once pleasurable, including sex
- Overeating or appetite loss
- Persistent sad, anxious, or "empty" feelings
- Thoughts of suicide, suicide attempts

It is extremely important that you establish a relationship with a doctor **prior to** feeling sick so they can get to know you and your specific health issues as well as learn about your lysosomal storage disease.

How do you find and establish a good relationship with a physician?

Asking your friends and your parents' friends and coworkers for recommendations is often a good start to finding a doctor. You will need to find out if the physician is 'in-network' or 'out-of-network' with your insurance company. (More information on this issue in the useful yellow box on page 11) This approach should work well for primary care physicians and some specialists. To manage your overall LSD care, we recommend working with a Lysosomal Storage Disease Treatment Center. You can find these centers on the Emory LSDC's link at (http://genetics.emory.edu/lsdcenters) or by contacting a patient support group. For example, the National Gaucher Foundation (NGF) (www.gaucherdisease.org) has a Treatment Center Locator on its website. Here you will find names, addresses and phone numbers for doctors who specialize in Gaucher disease. You might be surprised to find a center close to you.

1. http://yourtotalhealth.ivillage.com/when-call-doctor.html?pageNum=3

Make a List. You should bring a list of questions with you to each of your visits with the physician, genetic counselor, and/or nurse, so you won't forget to ask a question important to you. Some important questions might include:

- Do you follow other patients with a lysosomal storage disease? Although this is a good question to ask, a 'yes' is not essential to making your final decision. It is important to remember that most physicians will not have much experience treating patients with a lysosomal storage disease. That is OK. The important personality trait you need in your healthcare provider is that they are willing to learn about your condition and work with your healthcare team to manage your LSD.

- If I am concerned about a particular pain or ache, will I be able to reach you and/or your nurse in a timely manner? What is the best way to do that?

- Do you use email to talk to patients?

If you feel good about the visit, feel the physician is interested in learning about you and your disease, and feel s/he is accessible, go with your instincts. Make sure that you have the best number to reach the office staff with you at all times. Program it under emergency numbers in your smart phone, laptop, or other electronic device. You should also have the phone number for your main health care providers programmed into your contacts list.

The second biggest recommendation to address your worries about who to contact when you are ill is to understand your condition, its treatment and on-going research. The more you know and understand your disease, the better prepared you will be to determine whether you should call your doctor's office or head straight to the emergency room.

Where can I go to find the most up-to-date information on my lysosomal storage disease?

The best way to find current information on your LSD is by talking to your local lysosomal storage disease center (LSDC) or genetics doctor. They usually have a wide variety of information for you and your other doctors. Another great resource is a support group for your specific condition. They often have easy-to-understand descriptions about your disease and can point you to other great information. Beyond these resources, most companies that offer therapies for LSDs will offer a disease summary or monograph that includes the fundamental basics of the disease, signs and symptoms, recommended schedule of assessments and clinical trial data. You can call the company and request such materials. Be sure to ask for two copies - one for you and one for your new physician. Understanding your disease allows you to take charge of your disease vs. allowing the disease to take charge of you. Handy links to LSDCs, support groups, and companies that treat LSDs can be found on the Emory LSDC website at www.genetics.emory.edu/LSD.

Why Do I Care if My Doctor is In-Network?

In-Network: A doctor who works closely with your insurance company, which means you pay less money for your doctor visits, test, etc.

Out-of-Network: A doctor who may accept your insurance, but does not work as closely with your insurance company. This means you pay more money for your medical care.

Why you should look at in-network doctors first: **It costs you less money!!**

3. I'm worried about managing my own treatment.

"Everybody makes mistakes every now and then. Once I was in the middle of exams and TOTALLY forgot that I had to get my infusion. When I remembered, I felt like a total fool and was so embarrassed. It took a day or two, but when I finally called <my genetic counselor> she told me what I might expect due to a missed infusion and we figured out a plan to get my next infusion in time for my next game. No harm, no foul. They didn't call the health police on me or send me back to the minor leagues."

Mike, an 18-year-old living with Gaucher disease

One of the biggest concerns teens have as they transition to adulthood is the responsibility of figuring out how to get ERT without the help of a parent. In many instances, a team has been working behind the scenes helping guide the process along. This team is most likely still in place. The team may consist of a physician, a genetic counselor, a nurse, and a case manager from the state, your insurance company, or the company that manufactures the drug. This team will help you, but you have to start asking the questions.

Here are some questions that you should start asking well before you leave the house and set off for college, a new job, a new city or your own place:

1. Does my new insurance cover my treatments? Do I have home care benefits (if this is an option you would like to explore and it has been cleared by your physician)?
2. Who will supply my drug and do I have their contact name and number?
3. Where will the drug be delivered? Do all the supplies come with the drug?
4. If you are on ERT: Where do I store ERT? Let's answer that question right here! Unless stated otherwise, enzyme replacement therapy should be stored in the refrigerator (2-8° C or 36-46 ° F).
5. How do I schedule my infusion appointments and what do I do when I get there?

The answers to many of these questions depend on your treatment plan and where you receive your care. If you are treated through ERT the location can make a large difference in how you proceed. If you are receiving your infusions at the local hospital, ask whether your appointment(s) should be scheduled with a central appointment desk or if you can schedule your next appointment right there with the nurse. A great tip from Trudi Holbrook, an infusion nurse at the Emory University Lysosomal Storage Disease Center, is to bring a calendar with you to each infusion to help schedule your next infusion appointment.

If you have a home care nurse, it is very important to remember to be there on the day of your infusion. It's easy to forget with friends, classes and/or work delays. Set up a system that works for everyone. Touching base the day before to be sure everyone has the appointment on his or her schedule is always a good idea.

Depending on your infusion location, your ERT medication may not be mixed before your IV is started. This can cause a time delay. Some enzymes take longer than others due to the number of vials. Ask the nurse or coordinating health care provider how to minimize time delays

The amount of time needed to infuse your enzyme is calculated based on your dose or amount of ERT you receive. The faster you give the infusion, the more likely you are to have a reaction. If you think the infusion is too long, review this with your doctor and/or nurse. Some infusions (i.e. Fabrazyme) can be sped up over time.

Bring a book, computer, iPod or work with you, as there may be downtime. Build this into your schedule and try and use this time as best you can. Catching up on reading, writing, or even sleep can make the time go by more quickly!

4. I'm worried that my nurse will administer ERT differently than I'm used to and I won't know how to talk to her/him.

"Don't be scared to ask questions about treatments. If you are uncomfortable with a treatment, let the healthcare providers know, so it doesn't get MORE uncomfortable. It's your body."

Hannah, a 16-year-old living with MPSVI

One of the most important relationships you will have is your relationship with your infusion nurse. Whether he or she is a homecare nurse or a nurse in an infusion center, the more open and honest you are with her/him, the better your relationship will be.

Nurses are very adept at treating all sorts of diseases and conditions, but their approaches may be slightly different. Some nurses are more comfortable using one brand of an IV, while others prefer a different brand. Some infusion centers may recommend that all their patients have port-a-cath implanted for drug administration while others prefer peripheral access.

Let's take a look at the following story:
Sue was used to Betty, her homecare nurse, coming to the house every two weeks to administer her ERT. Everything was great. One day, however, Betty was out sick and a new nurse came. Sue soon realized that the new nurse was not doing things at all the same way Betty did. For starters, she didn't mix the drug at the counter where Betty always mixed it. She also didn't start the IV in Sue's left hand, where Sue wanted it.

How might Sue talk to her new nurse so that nobody's feelings get hurt and everyone is happy with the results?

"Hi! Thanks for coming. I know there's more than one way to do this and you probably do things a little different than Betty. Before we get started, though, can we talk about what I'm used to and what's worked well in the past?"

Or, if your new nurse has already started doing things differently:

"Hi! Thanks so much for coming. Do you mind if we use my right hand instead of my left for the IV? It's more comfortable for me that way. Thanks."

Use the blank space below to write what you might say to a new nurse about mixing your drug in a different location than usual.

_____

_____

_____

_____

One suggestion might sound like this:

"If it's OK with you, can we mix the drug here? This has been a great place to mix it in the past."

Let's assume you are planning on using the time during your infusion to work on a term paper. How might you approach the subject with a new nurse?

"Would you mind looking at my left-hand first? I have a term paper that I really need to work on today. Thank you so much!"

Unlike many drugs, enzyme replacement therapy is not very harmful to your veins, so nurses used to infusing drugs for cancer or other diseases may be surprised to learn that, after all this time, you still don't have a port or that you're using the same hand for access and treatment. This is where having basic knowledge about your disease and its treatment will come in handy and you may have to provide a little basic education about ERT to your new nurse.

Nurses, doctors, and for that matter parents are not mind readers. It is important that you share your concerns. Go with your instincts! Keep in mind that YOU are in charge of your medical care and can make requests that should be honored unless it is harmful to you or puts others at risk.

Let's review another scenario:

Sam never missed an infusion and knew the routine pretty well. When the drug arrived from the pharmacy and was about to be hung on the IV pole, however, Sam noticed that it was in a tiny bag of fluid — not the usual 250 cc bag he was used to seeing. Could that be right? What would YOU do? At this moment, do you know how much fluid your enzyme should be mixed in?

In this particular scenario, Sam was correct to question the amount of fluid. Indeed, there had been an error in mixing the product. Go with your instincts! Ask questions. If something doesn't feel right, it may not be! Be polite, but firm when asking your questions. Again, this is where understanding your own treatment will serve you well.

5. I'm concerned about making my own doctor's appointments and transitioning to adult medicine.

"OK, so I still went to my pediatrician until I turned 21! I was so comfortable with her, even though I felt a little silly sitting in the waiting room. It took a little bit of doctor shopping, but I found a great "grown-up" doctor and now I don't have to be examined with a giraffe stethoscope!"

Maria, a 22-year-old living with Pompe disease

Managing your medical information often means making your doctors appointments, arriving on time, filling out medical forms and having a place to keep your records so you can be as accurate as possible when answering questions. The Children's Hospital of Wisconsin has the following steps to offer:

- Ask your pediatric primary/specialty care doctor to recommend an adult primary/specialty care doctor for you.

- Check your healthcare insurance policy to make sure the adult doctor recommended by your pediatrician is approved by your insurance plan. [Hint: this may be described in your policy as the doctor's being "in-network" (i.e. approved by your insurance plan) or "out-of-network" (i.e. may not be approved by your insurance plan!)] Not everyone's insurance plan is the same, so be sure to check your own policy rather than relying on someone else's! If the doctor is not approved by your insurance plan, go back to your pediatric doctor and ask for another recommendation from among those doctors who are approved in network.

- Meet with the new adult primary care doctor before making the decision whether or not s/he is the right person to manage your health. Think of it as an interview. The relationship between patient and physician is very important. Each patient may be looking for something different in a physician (e.g. can you email them?) and that's OK. Whether or not a doctor is right for you will become obvious as you interview them. Bring a list of questions with you to make it a more meaningful and effective visit.

- Be sure to interview a potential adult doctor *before you feel sick*. You will not have the time or energy to interview someone once you are ill!

- Some doctors have on-line scheduling systems for appointments and obtaining lab results. If this is an important perk for you, ask possible doctors about this option.

What information will your adult doctors need?

- Copy of your transition plan (You will help develop this as a part of *Transitions: Managing Your Own Healthcare* in Chapter 9.)

- Copy of a clinical summary. A clinical summary is a document that covers your important medical information, both past and present. It introduces you to your adult primary and specialty care providers and helps them begin to take over your healthcare. Typically you can request a clinical summary from the pediatric physician who currently manages the majority of your care. An example of a clinical summary can be found in Chapter 9.

- Copies of your medical records. Providing contact information for someone on both your pediatric primary and specialty care teams is important to your new doctors if any of your medical information needs to be clarified. There are records release forms you have to sign at the doctor's office to give your permission to share your medical records.

6. I'm concerned about insurance coverage & doctors' bills.

Well, you're not alone on this one. Insurance coverage seems to be one of the biggest concerns expressed by nearly all teens and young adults, with or without a lysosomal storage disease. With ongoing changes in healthcare reform, it's imperative that you understand the basics, know where to turn to get answers, and most of all, be proactive! It's important to remember that you don't need to be an insurance expert; you just need to know your resources and where to turn for help.

First, the fast answer to the question, *What if I get a bill from my doctor, hospital, clinic, etc?*

1. DO NOT IGNORE IT! The faster you take care of it, the less you may owe.

2. If the bill appears to be correct, pay it. Make sure that you keep careful notes about what you have paid for which service. Keep copies of the bill, so you can compare them later. Remember that most insurance plans have co-pays or deductibles that you may be responsible for at the beginning of every year. Talk over your responsibilities with your case manager at the end of every year so you are prepared for the bills in January and know what is correct to pay. In some cases a nonprofit organization such as Patient Services Incorporated or a copay assistance plan from the pharmaceutical company may help pay for your deductible or copay. Learn how to sign up for these programs, find out what the limitations of the programs are, and know where to send bills and documentation.

3. If you have questions about a bill, you should call the phone number on the bill to find out more information. Do not just leave a message. You must talk to a person if you want answers. Questions you should ask include:

   a. What is the total amount of the bill I owe? Make sure you have a copy of the bill to review during the call. With a copy of the bill, you can make sure you are talking about the same charges and calling the right number. If you need another copy of your doctors' bills, you may need to request them from the doctors' office, a billing office, or another facility.

b. What are the dates of office visits and other services that are charged to this bill? These are designed to make sure that the bill is accurate and that you received the services that are being charged to you.

c. If there is a bill, was it sent to your insurance company or other assistance organization?

d. If it was not sent to your insurance company, you need to ask them to send it to your insurance company. Make sure they have the right insurance information. Ask who to call and when to call to follow up — how many days?

e. Ask if anything went to collections. Collections means you have not paid your bill for a long time and they have sent the bill to another company to get the money from you. If a bill goes to collections, you need to take care of it immediately or it will negatively affect your credit. If it affects your credit, you will have a hard time buying a house, a car or other things.

f. Ask the name of the person you spoke to on the phone and write it down, along with the day and time that you called. Make sure to take notes on what they tell you. Keep an ongoing log of phone calls for bills, so you can look at your phone record and say who you spoke to and what they told you. That way, you can refer back to the conversation if you get another bill from the same organization for the same date and service you called about before.

g. Don't forget about it. Make sure the issue is resolved before you file it away. Ask for help from your parents, case manager, genetic counselor, etc., if things are not resolved in a month's time.

> An explanation of benefits (commonly referred to as an EOB form) is a paper statement sent by a health insurance company to a covered individual explaining what medical treatments and/or services were paid for on their behalf. The statement will tell you why a particular medical charge wasn't covered and what your expected payment to the doctor or hospital will be. It is often tagged with the line "This is Not a Bill."

Now the long answer: Insurance!

Insurance coverage is vitally important, not just for coverage for your treatment but for your overall health and well-being. Below are scenarios concerning healthcare coverage for two young adults in different situations. You many not know how to answer their questions now, but hopefully as you read through this section, you'll have a better understanding of their individual options.

Example 1: *Jane is 18 years of age and recently found out she has LAL-deficiency. She is about to graduate from high school and has been accepted to a state university in the fall to start college. What type of insurance is available to her?*

Example 2: *Mike is 19 years of age and excited about his new job at Home Depot. Mike has MPS Type II. What are his insurance options?*

The landscape of healthcare coverage in the United States is changing constantly and it can be difficult to keep up with the latest policies. The following information is current as of 2013. If there is ever a doubt in your mind where the law stands, never hesitate to contact your own insurance company directly, or ask someone in your healthcare management team — a parent, counselor, case manager, etc. — to help you research the answer.

The 2010 Affordable Care Act

According to USA.gov, the 2010 Affordable Care Act put in place health insurance reforms. Although some new provisions are already in place, most changes will take effect by 2014. The following provisions may be relevant to you:

- Expanded coverage for young adults, allowing them to stay on their parents' plan until they turn 26 years old or can get their own insurance through a job

- Providing access to insurance for uninsured Americans with pre-existing conditions

The U.S. government's HealthCare.gov website has a special page dedicated to Young Adult Coverage that addresses criteria for young adult coverage under the new system. The webpage can be accessed at: http://www.healthcare.gov/law/features/choices/young-adult-coverage/index.html

Another particularly valuable resource may be the Young Adult and the Affordable Care Act Factsheet, available at: http://www.healthcare.gov/news/factsheets/2011/08/young-adults.html

Just like someone with diabetes or any other health ailment, as an individual with a lysosomal storage disease, you qualify as having a pre-existing condition.

> A pre-existing condition is a health problem that exists before you apply for a health insurance policy or enroll in a new health plan.

Some of the new laws associated with the 2010 Affordable Care Act are aimed at securing healthcare coverage for individuals under the age of 19 with a pre-existing condition. To find out whether this information might be relevant to you, you can visit: http://www.healthcare.gov/law/features/rights/childrens-pre-existing-conditions/index.html

The implementation timeline of the 2010 Affordable Care Act is a great resource to help figure out which parts of the bill have been implemented at any given date: http://www.healthcare.gov/law/timeline/index.html

An Overview of Health Insurance Coverage

The following is meant to serve as an overview to health insurance coverage as it stands at publication. Please note that as healthcare reform advances, changes in the law may replace information contained within this module. The "Find Insurance Options" at http://finder.healthcare.gov/ can help set you on your way.

Types of Health Insurance Plans

There are a number of different plans available for those looking for health insurance coverage:

- An individual plan, if the coverage is just for yourself
- If you have a partner, you can opt for joint coverage
- If you have a family, you can opt for family coverage

With most comprehensive health insurance plans, you can expect benefits such as:

- Physician care
- Hospital care (as an in-patient or out-patient)
- Dental and Vision
- Prescription (Medication) benefits
- Surgery and other major medical benefits

You Get What You Pay For

As with any other type of insurance (e.g. auto), the more comprehensive the plan, the more the premium (the amount you have to pay) may cost. It is very important to read the policy completely before committing, as many health insurance plans contain a lot of exclusions (items that aren't covered). You may find that you are not covered for certain problems or in certain situations that you know will be important for you. As you have a pre-existing condition, you may also find that this is not covered under the policy for one year. You should also know if the policy covers genetic testing or pregnancy/delivery costs.

If you have any concerns about the policy you are thinking of buying, you should address your concerns with a representative from the insurance company, a case manager, and/or your Human Resources (HR) partner at your or your parents' job before you make your decision.

Private and Public Sources for Coverage

Health insurance coverage is provided by a wide array of public and private sources.

Public sources include:

- Medicare
- Medicaid
- Federal and state employee health plans
- Military
- Veterans Administration

Example of Publicly Offered Insurance

Medicaid and Medicare are examples of government offered (public) insurance. In most cases, a young adult with a disability will remain on Medicaid or Medicare. As an example, in Georgia, PeachCare and Katie Beckett both provide Medicaid coverage until you turn 19 years old. It is important, however, that you and your parent/guardian discuss the requirements for maintaining government insurance for an adult with a disability with your caseworker before you turn 18 years old. The Supplemental Security Income (SSI) program pays benefits to disabled adults and children who have limited income and resources. Applying for SSI on-line is free of charge by going to www.ssa.gov or calling toll-free 1-800-772-1213.

Example of Private Insurance

Private health insurance coverage is provided primarily through benefit plans sponsored by employers – about 162 million people are insured through employer-sponsored health insurance. People without access to employer-sponsored insurance (i.e. whose jobs do not provide insurance or who are unemployed) may obtain health insurance on their own, usually through the individual health insurance market. In some cases, health insurance may also be available to individuals through professional associations or similar groups.

Let's Take a Closer Look at Private Health Insurers

Commercial Health Insurers Commercial health insurers (also referred to as indemnity insurers) are generally organized as stock companies (owned by stockholders) or as mutual insurance companies (owned by their policyholders). A prime example is Aetna, a stock company.

Blue Cross Blue Shield Plans Historically, many of these plans were organized as not-for-profit organizations under special state laws by state hospital (Blue Cross) and state medical (Blue Shield) associations. Today, many Blue Cross and Blue Shield plans operate as commercial insurance companies. There are still a few states, however, in which they continue to operate under special state laws and have special requirements to accept individuals for health insurance on a more lenient basis than is applied to other types of insurers.

Health Maintenance Organizations (HMOs) HMOs are a more recent addition to the world of healthcare insurance plans. HMOs operate both as insurers (meaning they spread healthcare costs across the people enrolled in their plan) and as healthcare providers (meaning they directly provide or arrange for the necessary healthcare for the people enrolled in their plan).

The popularity of HMOs has grown over the years because they are often the least expensive with regard to monthly premiums. One of the drawbacks, however, is that certain restrictions may apply to keep costs down, so you will want to be very careful when examining the care provided by any policy before you buy it. You will want to know up front if enzyme replacement therapy is covered. In addition, HMOs usually designate specific healthcare providers you are allowed to visit. In the event of an emergency, if you visit an unapproved provider, you may be left to pick-up the entire tab yourself. Examples of state-licensed HMOs include Kaiser Permanente and Harvard Pilgrim.

High-Deductible Plan A high-deductible health plan (HDHP) is a health insurance plan with lower premiums and higher deductibles than a traditional health plan. Being covered by an HDHP is also a requirement for having a health savings account. Some HDHP plans also offer additional "wellness" benefits, provided before a deductible is paid. High-deductible health plans are a form of catastrophic coverage, intended to cover catastrophic illnesses. This is usually not a good option for individuals with a chronic health condition like a LSD.

Fee-for-Services Health Insurance As its name implies, fee-for-services health insurance is a basic indemnity policy.

In short, with fee-for-services health insurance, you submit a claim whenever you go to see a doctor or get medical treatment and your health insurance provider deducts the cost from your pre-agreed health insurance sum. The upside of fee-for-services health insurance is that you can visit any healthcare provider you want and then make a claim – although you should still read the health insurance policy carefully, as some types of treatment may not be covered. Once again, it's always going to be a good idea to make sure your treatment, like ERT, is a covered benefit before you buy any insurance policy!

With every upside, there is a downside. The major downside of fee-for-services health insurance is the cost. Unlike other types of health insurance, which came on the market after fee-for-services, monthly premiums in fee-for-service insurance can be high. The only way to reduce the higher premiums (the amount you pay every month) is to increase your deductibles (the amount you pay if you actually go to the doctor). However, you want to think carefully before increasing your deductibles, as this can lead to your being left with a hefty bill if you need hospital treatment.

Other types of healthcare insurance In response to the high cost of fee-for-services healthcare insurance and the restrictions of HMOs regarding which doctors you can see, other types of healthcare insurance were created. Among these are Preferred Provider Organizations (PPOs). Like HMOs, PPOs do have a network of particular doctors you are encouraged to visit; however, you are sometimes allowed to see doctors outside of that network if you don't mind paying a slightly higher percentage of the cost (e.g. you might pay 30% rather than 20% of the doctor's bill). How much more you pay depends on the particular healthcare policy you have.

Flexible Spending Accounts A flexible spending account (FSA), also known as a flexible spending arrangement, is one of a number of tax-advantaged financial accounts that can be set up through your job. An FSA allows an employee to set aside a portion of earnings to pay for qualified medical expenses. Money is deducted from an employee's pay into an FSA and is not subject to payroll taxes, resulting in substantial payroll tax savings. One significant disadvantage to using an FSA is that funds not used by the end of the plan year are lost to the employee, known as the "use it or lose it" rule. Please note, FSA funds can't be used to buy over-the-counter medications.

Health Savings Accounts These are medical savings accounts available to taxpayers in the United States who are enrolled in a high-deductible health plan (HDHP). The funds contributed to an account are not subject to federal income tax at the time of deposit. Unlike a flexible spending account (FSA), funds roll over and accumulate year to year if not spent. HSAs are owned by the individual. HSA funds may currently be

Indemnity: a contractual agreement made between different parties to compensate for any damages or losses

used to pay for qualified medical expenses at any time without federal tax liability or penalty. They can't be used to buy over-the-counter medications.

Summing it all up

So, if you are looking for health insurance, there are many options in the public as well as the private sector. Please make sure you give special thought to buying health insurance and make sure that you are not one of the 40 million Americans today walking around with no healthcare insurance! As comforting as it might be to keep alive the eternal hope that your lysosomal storage disease is going to go away, a cure has not been discovered yet, only treatment – and getting that treatment means having good health insurance!

A Word of Advice

It is very important to check with your parents' insurance company before you turn 18 years old to verify the length and terms of your coverage under your parents' family plan. Maintaining insurance coverage with no lapse or gaps in coverage is very important, as having time without insurance can cause a delay in getting new coverage. When in doubt, check with your case manager to help determine your coverage benefits. They are usually experts in their field and can give

you guidance, help you understand the policy and help you understand the financial responsibility associated with the policy. If your parent has always been the one to make contact with your case manager, now is the time for you to call and introduce yourself. Available resources are listed under RESOURCES in Chapter 8 of this learning module.

Healthcare guidelines that began in 2010

New changes in the law that began in 2010 are a great help to teens with medical problems. Insurance companies are no longer able to write policies that refuse to pay for a particular medical condition. However, they can still deny new individual policies to children in poor health. So, when in doubt, always ask!

Also new as of 2010, the law requires all health insurance plans to maintain dependent coverage for children until they turn 26 years of age! What's the effect on your wallet? The good news is a law is under consideration that would prevent insurers and employers from raising the cost if young adults remain on their parent's policy. Furthermore, the rules state that premiums (the amount you pay each month) must remain the same, regardless of the age of the teen.

I worry about exhausting a lifetime maximum on my insurance policy.

One big concern with enzyme replacement therapy is that it is so expensive and could easily exhaust a 2-million-dollar lifetime max while you are still young. Effective for health plan years beginning on or after September 23, 2010, insurance companies are prohibited from imposing lifetime dollar limits on essential benefits. New guidelines will keep insurance companies from putting lifetime dollar limits or maximums on coverage - and from canceling policies, except in cases of fraud. However, it is important to pay attention to details. While lifetime limits are prohibited, annual limits are still effective until 2014.

Let's return to our two scenarios and see if we now better understand the insurance options available.

Jane is 18 years of age and recently found out she has LAL deficiency. She is about to graduate from high school and has been accepted to a state university in the fall to start college. What type of insurance is available to her?

Off to college: *Currently, two options are available to Jane as she is entering college; she can remain on her family plan or enroll in the college-sponsored plan. Pre-planning is important so as not to interrupt her enzyme replacement therapy*

schedule. A third option may also exist for Jane. Assuming she can work part-time, some employers offer health benefits for part-time employees.

Mike is 19 years of age and excited about his new job at Home Depot. Mike has MPS Type II. What are his insurance options?

State Funded Plans: *Mike may be under a state funded plan that ends when he turns 19 years old. His new job at Home Depot may offer insurance coverage; however, there might be an open enrollment period with Home Depot as to when he can apply/change his coverage benefits. It would be wise for him to check into these open enrollment periods. His case manager or the Human Resources benefits office at Home Depot would be good places for him to start getting the information he needs.*

In summary, as you finish your teen years and transition into a young adult, various types of insurance options will become available to you and some may no longer be an option due to your age. Navigating the insurance waters doesn't have to be difficult - there are many resources available to help you. It is very important that every teen and/or young adult with medical needs obtain insurance, whether it is through a public plan, a private plan, or community programs.

My Health Insurance

Exercise: *Start by answering the following questions:*

Do I have health insurance? ☐ **Yes** ☐ **No**

Is my health insurance through my parents? ☐ **Yes** ☐ **No**

Who is my health insurance provider? _____
(name of company or public program)

Will my health insurance change when I turn 18 years old, go to school or get a job? ☐ **Yes** ☐ **No**

Knowing the answers to these questions is the first step towards making sure you have the health insurance you need. If you're not sure, ask your parents, your doctor, and/or your health insurance provider.

Now, write down one name, one phone number and/or one website where you can go for help in understanding your insurance coverage.

Name: _____

Phone: _____

Website: _____

Turning to the Web for Help

Social Security Administration: Not just for the old

You may think Social Security is just for old retired people. In reality, however, the Social Security Administration serves teens and young adults too. The Social Security Administration is accessible online (www.socialsecurity.gov) and is a must-read website if you have a disability and need to know about coverage. This is a user-friendly site that we highly recommend you review with your parent(s) and/or your case manager.

Social Security (SS) and Supplemental Security Income (SSI) disability programs are the largest of several Federal programs that provide assistance to people with disabilities. The Social Security Administration administers both of these programs. While the two programs are different in many ways, only individuals who have a disability and meet certain medical criteria qualify for benefits under either program.

How do I know if I qualify for SS Disability benefits? What is the first step?

The above mentioned website will help guide you. To apply for Social Security benefits, call toll-free 1-800-772-1213. More information can also be obtained at www.ssa.gov.

Children's Health Insurance Program (CHIP)

Originally created in 1997, the Children's Health Insurance Program (CHIP) is a state and federal partnership that provides low-cost health insurance for children under the age of 19 in families which make too much money to qualify for Medicaid but still cannot afford private health insurance. States have considerable flexibility in establishing income eligibility rules for CHIP, but in general, children enrolling in the program must not have any other insurance.

Within federal guidelines, each state designs its own individual CHIP program, including income criteria, benefit packages, payment levels, and administrative procedures. All states are required, however, to cover routine check-ups, immunizations, dental, inpatient and outpatient hospital care, and laboratory and x-ray services. Preventive medical care must also be provided, at no cost to the family; however, premiums and other cost sharing may be required for other medical services.

InsureKidsNow.gov

www.insurekidsnow.gov also has many resources and is another must-read link if your family earns too much income to qualify for Medicaid but cannot afford private health insurance.

CHIP in 50 States

Every state and U.S. Territory operates a CHIP program, although many states have unique names for their programs. For example, in Georgia, it is called PeachCare. Click on the map at www.InsureKidsNow.gov to learn more about your state's programs.

Each state also has different rules about Medicaid eligibility and services. If you or someone in your family needs healthcare, you should apply for Medicaid even if you aren't sure if you qualify and get a qualified caseworker in your state to help look at your situation.

InsureKidsNow.gov has a Medicaid program in your state (http://www.InsureKidsNow.gov/) – or you can make a free call to 1-877-KIDS NOW (1-877-543-7669) to discuss your situation with someone from your state.

Extra help for individuals with LSDs

Individuals with LSDs may qualify for programs that help pay copays, deductibles, or other LSD related healthcare expenses. These programs may include Patient Services Incorporated (PSI), NORD, PANF, or pharmaceutical co-pay assistance plans. Talk to your healthcare provider or case manager to determine what programs you may qualify for and how to apply.

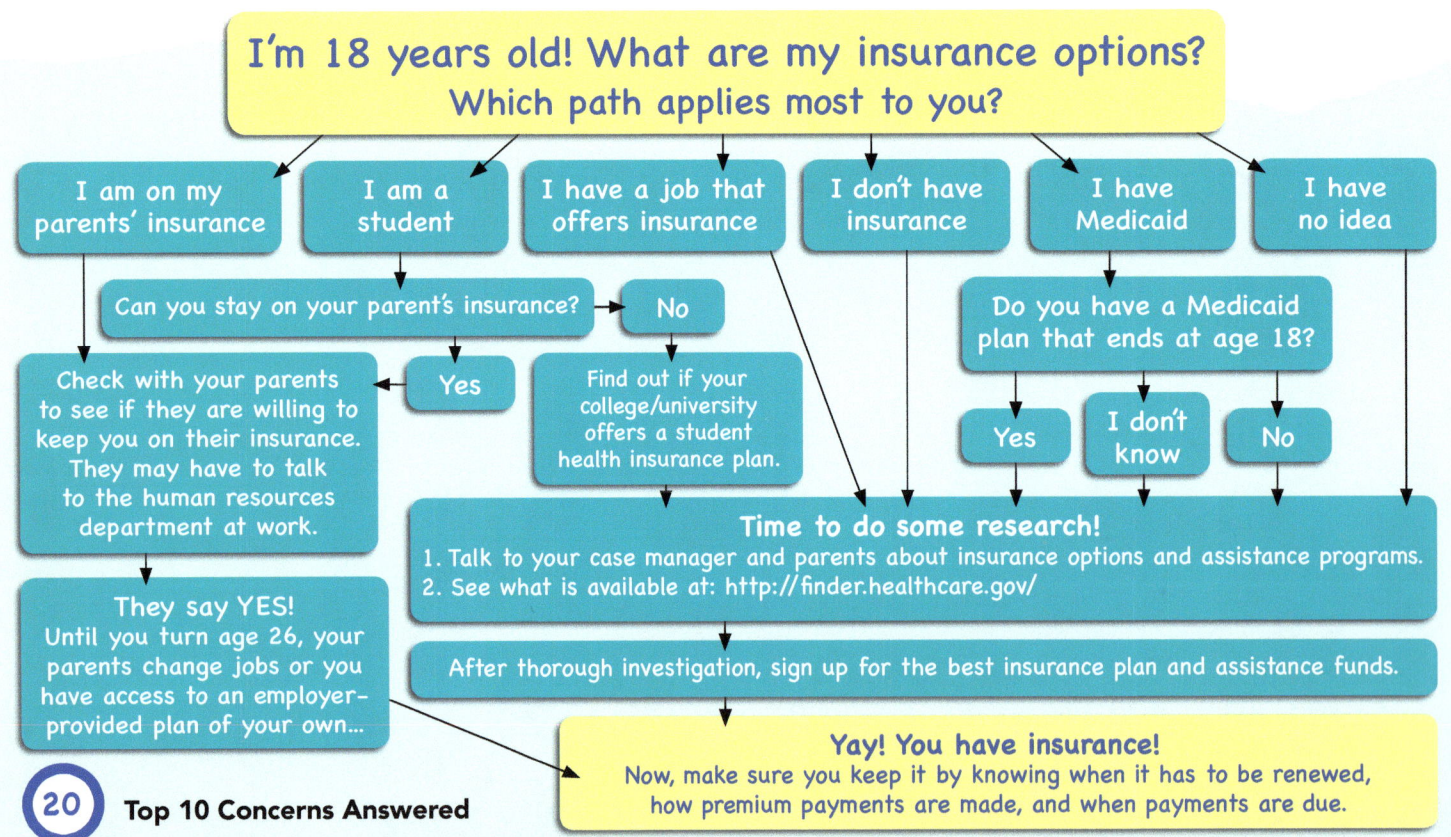

I'm 18 years old! What are my insurance options? Which path applies most to you?

- I am on my parents' insurance
- I am a student
- I have a job that offers insurance
- I don't have insurance
- I have Medicaid
- I have no idea

Can you stay on your parent's insurance?

- No
- Yes

Check with your parents to see if they are willing to keep you on their insurance. They may have to talk to the human resources department at work.

Find out if your college/university offers a student health insurance plan.

Do you have a Medicaid plan that ends at age 18?

- Yes
- I don't know
- No

Time to do some research!
1. Talk to your case manager and parents about insurance options and assistance programs.
2. See what is available at: http://finder.healthcare.gov/

They say YES! Until you turn age 26, your parents change jobs or you have access to an employer-provided plan of your own...

After thorough investigation, sign up for the best insurance plan and assistance funds.

Yay! You have insurance! Now, make sure you keep it by knowing when it has to be renewed, how premium payments are made, and when payments are due.

7. I'm concerned about getting transportation to appointments and infusions.

"I don't drive. Don't have a license. Never have, probably never will. I still get to my doctor's office. Remember, it's not your responsibility to drive, but it is your responsibility to find a ride."

Miranda, a 20-year-old living with MPS IV (Morquio)

Many teens living with a lysosomal storage disease don't have a driver's license, either because of a limitation or because they simply choose not to have one. The availability of public transportation (i.e. trains, buses) is an option in some places, but not in others. Nonetheless, you must make arrangements to get to and from your appointments and infusions, usually well in advance.

So what transportation options are available to me?
Many states have a *Medicaid Non-Emergency Transportation* **(NET) program** for those Medicaid members who need rides to medical care or services. In a search engine, type in Medicaid Transportation Services to see what's available in your state. Theses rides must be organized in advance, often 3-7 days before your appointment.

In Georgia, for example, there are five NET regions serving the state. You can get further information by calling 1-866-211-0950 or going to www.dch.Georgia.gov. Please check into the amount of time you will need to schedule in advance for a ride and if there are any restrictions on types of appointments you can use the transportation to reach.

If your infusions are scheduled at a local hospital, you can also call the main hospital number to ask if they have available transportation services.

8. I'm concerned that when I can make my own medical decisions I won't want to do my infusions.

Yes, you do get to make your own medical decisions now. That means that, as an adult, you do have more freedom and flexibility. Technically, you could choose not to get your infusions anymore. However, when asked what's most important to them about their health, most people say they want to feel as good as they can each day. They want optimal health.

Here's the deal. You have a lysosomal storage disease. You also have treatment available that people didn't have many years ago (in some cases, can't even get now!). Some countries, to this day, still don't have access to enzyme replacement therapy or other treatment options.

Allow us to share a story with you. Gaucher disease is a lysosomal storage disease in which a missing enzyme causes storage of a particular substance to build up in your bones (if you have Gaucher disease, you should know this substance is called glucocerebroside). Prior to ERT, when you attended a patient meeting, it looked more like an orthopedic meeting, with walkers, canes, and even wheelchairs in every corner. With the discovery of ERT, we began to see a totally different picture emerge. Now at patient meetings, the focus is more on quality of life issues, sports and camps for teens. Gone are most of the wheelchairs, canes, and walkers. The change didn't occur without enzyme replacement therapy (ERT). And it didn't occur due to non-adherence (missing infusions).

We get it! We hear quite often that people want to take a break from their infusions. Do you know anyone with high blood pressure or high cholesterol? They have to take their medications sometimes three and four times a day and yet they say they don't feel any different. You know what happens when they stop their medications? That's right, blood pressure and cholesterol levels creep back up and cause big problems. The same holds true with enzyme replacement therapy. You may not feel much of a difference on ERT, but you need it to keep from getting sicker as your disease progresses. Sometimes stabilizing the disease is the primary goal. Taking even one step backwards carries risk. Without ERT, substrate builds up and the burden of disease increases, often silently and without you being aware of it.

Enzyme replacement therapy can only fix so much. Once the disease process has gone too far there is no turning back. All of the enzyme in the world can't make a flattened hipbone round again, as in the case of Gaucher disease. It can't make a scarred Fabry kidney function normally again. It can't undo a stroke. Keep in mind that if and when they find a "cure" for LSDs you want to be healthy enough for it to work for **you**.

Yeah, but I have to get infusions every week or every two weeks. Yes you do. That's how it works for now. Great advances in research are being made that may allow you to receive ERT less frequently or even take a pill instead. At 18 years old, you have the right to be a part of clinical research. There may be trials that are looking at alternate treatments or dosing right now. You can find out about new clinical trials by going to www.clinicaltrials.gov or asking your healthcare provider about studies you may qualify to join.

If you are thinking about missing infusions, you need to talk to your parent(s), physicians, and/or a knowledgeable health care provider. Together you can determine exactly why you want to stop therapy and you can address this together.

It might be a good idea to talk to your doctor, genetic counselor, and other people your own age who have been there before. Depending on the reason for discontinuing therapy, there are usually options to help. For example, if you really don't like getting stuck every two weeks, placement of a port-a-cath to help with IV access might make a difference. The use of a numbing cream at the access site might make a difference. There could be home care benefits through your insurance plan, if transportation is the key issue. Whatever your reason, there probably is a way to work with you and keep you on a schedule.

The Lysosomal Storage Disease Center of Emory University evaluated four patients who elected to go off infusion therapy. Karen Grinzaid, MS, CGC, lead author on the published paper, comments that, "Over time, everyone who stopped ERT, particularly children and young adults, experienced problems related to their Gaucher disease and required more aggressive therapy to get them back on course."[2]

9. I'm worried that I don't understand my disease or treatment well enough to get the best medical care and make good decisions.

Understanding your specific lysosomal storage disease is a very important aspect of your healthcare. The learning curve for beginning to understand your disease should begin at around 14 years of age. At this age, it is important to be able to verbalize what your particular lysosomal storage disease is with your teachers, doctors and other healthcare professionals. This may consist of a couple of short paragraphs that you can develop with the help of a genetic counselor or a patient care advocate/liaison from one of the companies offering treatment. It may sound something like this:

"My lysosomal storage disease is caused because I am missing an enzyme or have a reduced amount of a certain enzyme. As a result, my body is not able to break down a specific substance (a lipid) and stores it in various places in my body.

Just like kids with diabetes have to take insulin to replace what they don't have, I have to take pills every day to reduce the stuff (lipids) stored in my cells or get regular infusion to replace the missing enzyme.

It's really important that I take my medication or get my infusions on a regular schedule because once the lipid builds up to a certain point and causes irreversible damage, it's hard for any amount of enzyme to fix the problem."

At age 16, this paragraph should become more detailed and have more depth around the discussions with healthcare professionals. By age 18 to 21, you should have in-depth knowledge of your disease and treatment, on-going clinical research, and specialists that should be involved with your on-going care. Many of the patient organizations have social media, Facebook pages, buddy programs, and meetings for young adults. You may want to check them out and become an active participant.

One of the frustrations expressed by many adults is they seem to know more about their disease than their physicians. Remember, lysosomal storage diseases are relatively rare, occurring in around 1 in every 7700 live births. So, unless you are part of a big center, you may be the only patient a physician follows with your disease. However, if you are prepared to do a little work up front, you can help ease this transition. Find a physician who is willing to learn about your particular lysosomal storage disease. Are they open to connecting to a lysosomal storage disease center, even if it is not located in the same city? If so, work closely with them as they learn more about you and your LSD.

Many physicians participate in a LSD Registry or outcome study. Registries and outcome surveys are confidential databases that house information on thousands of patients from around the world with your specific lysosomal storage disease. Leading authorities in the field of lysosomal storage diseases usually govern them. The data gleaned from the Registry is there to help physicians provide a standard of care, even if they are managing only one or two patients. Ask your healthcare provider if you are already enrolled in your disease-specific Registry.

2. Karen A. Grinzaid, et al, Cessation of enzyme replacement therapy in Gaucher disease, Genetics in Medicine, November/December 2002, Vol. 4, No. 6

How might this condition affect my family? Could other family members have my condition?

One additional question you may have wondered about is whether or not your children, brothers, or sisters could also be affected by your genetic condition. The answer depends on which genetic condition is affecting you.

Cystinosis, Gaucher, a Glycoprotein condition, Krabbe, LAL deficiency, a MPS condition (EXCEPT MPSII), Pompe, or Tay Sachs

If you have **Cystinosis, Gaucher, a Glycoprotein condition, Krabbe, LAL deficiency, a MPS condition (EXCEPT MPSII), Pompe, or Tay Sachs** then your condition is passed down in an "autosomal recessive" manner. Autosomal recessive is one of several ways that a genetic trait, disorder, or condition can be passed down through families. Recessive means that two copies of an abnormal, nonworking gene must be present in order for the condition to develop. When a person has a recessive disease, in most cases, both of their parents have one copy of the nonworking gene and are unaffected "carriers" for the condition. Both parents must pass their nonworking copies of the gene to their child in order for the child to have the genetic condition. Carrier parents have a 1 in 4 chance of passing on both copies of the nonworking gene to each of their kids. That also means they have a 1 in 4 chance of passing on each of their working genes resulting in a completely healthy child who is not a carrier, and a 50% (1 in 2) chance of passing on one nonworking gene and one working gene resulting in a child who is a carrier but unaffected. In summary, your brothers and sisters have a 25% chance to have the same condition that you do, a 25% chance to be unaffected non-carriers, and a 50% chance to be an unaffected carrier for the condition.

Since you have the condition, you have two nonworking copies of the gene. This means that you will pass on one nonworking gene to each of your children. The chance for your child to be affected is based on the carrier status of your partner. If your partner has two working copies of the gene, then all (100%) of your kids together would be unaffected carriers. If your partner is a carrier of one nonworking copy of the gene, then 50% of your children would be unaffected carriers and 50% would be affected by your condition. If your partner has the same genetic condition that you have then 100% of your children would be affected by the same genetic condition affecting you.

Fabry Disease

If you are affected by **Fabry disease** then your condition is passed down in an "X-linked" manner. X-linked inheritance is one of several ways that a genetic trait, disorder, or condition can be passed down through families With X-linked inheritance the nonworking gene that causes the disease, like Fabry disease, is located on the X-chromosome. The X-chromosome is a special chromosome that, along with the Y-chromosome in men, helps determine our gender. Women have two X chromosomes and men have one X chromosome and one Y-chromosome. If a woman has Fabry disease, she has an X-chromosome with one nonworking gene for Fabry disease and one X-chromosome with a working gene. If she passes down the nonworking gene to her child, that child will have Fabry disease whether it is a boy or a girl. If she passes down the X-chromosome with the working gene, the child will NOT have Fabry disease. There is a 50% chance that she will pass down the working gene and a 50% chance that she will pass down the nonworking gene. A man with Fabry disease has one X-chromosome with a nonworking gene for Fabry. The Y-chromosome does not contain any genes for Fabry disease. For a man with Fabry disease, all of his daughters will have Fabry disease and none of his sons will be affected since he will pass down his Y-chromosome to all of his sons.

Mucopolysaccharidosis Type II (MPSII or Hunter Syndrome)

If you are affected by **Mucopolysaccharidosis Type II (MPSII or Hunter Syndrome),** then your condition is passed down in an "X-linked recessive" manner. X-linked recessive inheritance is one of several ways that a genetic trait, disorder, or condition can be passed down through families. The IDS gene, when it does not work, causes MPSII and is located on the X-chromosome Women have two X chromosomes and men only have one X chromosome. Most of the time, a woman with one nonworking copy of the IDS gene does not have signs or symptoms of MPSII and is considered a carrier. Rarely, a woman with one nonworking copy of the IDS gene will have signs or symptoms of MPSII, but this does not usually occur. If a woman has one nonworking copy of the IDS gene (whether a carrier or affected), there is a 50% chance that her sons will be affected by MPSII and typically a 50% chance her daughters will be unaffected carriers. If a man has MPSII, all of his daughters will have one nonworking copy of the IDS gene (and in the vast majority of cases would not have MPSII) and none of his sons will be affected.

Everyone living with a lysosomal storage disease will deal with it in a different way; from telling the world you have an LSD, for instance, to only letting immediate family members know. No matter what you choose, it is your personal decision and should be respected.

Understanding HIPAA

When you turn 18-years-old, your parents are no longer considered your legal guardians. The Health Insurance Portability and Accountability Act (HIPAA) of 1995 established national standards to protect individuals' medical records and other personal health information. This Act applies to health plans, healthcare clearinghouses and those healthcare providers that conduct certain healthcare transactions electronically.

In plain English: **your healthcare records are private between you and your healthcare provider**. If you would like your parents and/or case manager to be involved in your healthcare and advocate for you, you will have to sign a consent form. You can usually get this form from either your case manager or your physician's office.

According to the US Department of Health and Human Services, HIPAA requires appropriate safeguards to protect the privacy of your personal health information, and sets limits and conditions on the uses and disclosures of your information without your permission. The rule also gives you rights regarding your health information, including the right to examine and obtain a copy of your health records and to request corrections.

If you don't want anyone to know you are living with a lysosomal storage disease, we'd like you to consider exploring why you don't want anyone to know. You might be amazed to learn that there is someone else at work, on your college campus, or in your neighborhood with a lysosomal storage disease who would benefit from your friendship and having someone who understands what it is like to have a lifetime disease.

Sometimes sharing with just one supportive friend or family member can make all the difference. That person can help as a listening ear, a brainstorming partner, or support when you are sad or frustrated.

But I don't know how to tell my boyfriend, girlfriend, roommate, etc. that I have a lysosomal storage disease.

There isn't a right way or wrong way, a right time or wrong time to share with someone that you are living with a lysosomal storage disease. If you need help with how to start this conversation, ask your genetic counselor for suggestions. Your genetic counselor has a lot of experience with your disease and can be a big asset!

There are also groups which focus on particular LSDs and may have additional support options. If you have Gaucher, the **National Gaucher Foundation (NGF)** has a mentor program that may help point you in the right direction. You can access this program at www.gaucherdisease.org.

If you have Fabry, the **Fabry Support and Information Group (FSIG)** (http://www.fabry.org/) and **National Fabry Disease Foundation (NFDF)** (http://thenfdf.org/) also have resources to help. Don't forget to check Facebook for additional support pages related to these groups.

If you have MPS or Pompe, the **National MPS Society** (www.mpssociety.org) and the **Acid Maltase Deficiency Association (AMDA)** (www.amda-pompe.org) also have wonderful resources available to you.

If you have a glycoprotein condition, such as Mucolipidosis II/II or Mannosidosis, the **International Society for Mannosidosis & Related Diseases (ISMRD)** (http://www.ismrd.org/) is a great resource.

"I had told my new boyfriend that I had a health problem kinda like diabetes, but that I was lucky and could eat whatever I wanted and only had to get injections twice a month. That worked for then, but it wasn't quite right. I mean...I don't know if I want to have kids yet, but if I did, they could be affected by my Fabry disease. That's big. So, I just ignored it. Then, one day, he told me that he wanted to know more about it. ALL about it, because he really loves me and wants to know more. It was so sweet. So, I told him more and later, I took him to my genetics appointment to hear more. He didn't run away, he wasn't afraid. He told me he was so glad to know more. It helps him understand my "down days" when I don't want to do more than watch TV, even though I'm usually really active. He also now understand why I HAVE to get my treatments and can't skip to go to the lake"

Missy a 19-year-old living with Fabry disease.

A Place for Your Notes

Exercise: *Please use this section to write down notes to yourself or questions you may have:*

_____

_____

_____

_____

_____

_____

_____

_____

_____

_____

_____

_____

_____

_____

_____

_____

_____

_____

Chapter Four
Transition Timeline for Teens

Remember, you are not alone during this time when you are transitioning to independence. Your support team has been there for you during childhood and is still going to be with you during this time of transition. The timelines listed below are suggested ages for you and your support team to begin to consider specific needs and skill sets to prepare you for the day when you become fully independent.

Transition is a process, not an event. It should occur gradually with baby steps, building upon each step. One doesn't learn to read without knowing their ABCs. The same principle applies here. This transition will take time. Getting started at an early age is the best approach.

Age 14	Age 16	Age 18	Age 21
• Start to understand the basics of your disease and treatment • Statement of Transition Service Needs may be included in your IEP* *(see below for definition of IEP)*	• Able to communicate to teachers, physicians and others the basic aspects of your disease and treatment • Start to understand your medications and why you take each one • Start thinking about transitioning from pediatrics to internal medicine or family medicine	• Have the right to make all decisions about your healthcare • Understand your healthcare benefits, know who to call, and have an insurance card with you • Can register to vote • Can actively participate in research studies *(www.clinicaltrials.gov)* • Apply for SSI and reapply for Medical Assistance (MA) programs • Males need to register for selected services • May choose not to continue in school. Parent may override this decision until age 21	• Transition to adult healthcare providers should be complete and under your control unless special provisions are made • Should understand the basics of insurance, medical bills, filing claims, and settling disputes regarding claims • As of your 21st birthday, if you still qualify for medical assistance (MA), then limited adult MA services will begin

What is an IEP?

The Individualized Education Program (IEP) allows children and teens with delayed skills or other disabilities to get services and programs to help them succeed in the public school system. IEP services are free of charge to families.

The passage of the Individuals with Disabilities Education Act (IDEA 2004) allows parents of children with special needs to work with educators to develop a personalized plan to help their child succeed in the public school system. By 16 years of age, you have the right to be part of your IEP transition team.

Chapter Five
Ready to Manage Your Own Healthcare?

Knowing what you **don't know** is as important as knowing what you **do know**. So, let's do a **baseline assessment** to figure out how ready you are **right now** to manage your own healthcare. The following tool will help you figure out where your own gaps are in terms of managing your own healthcare. Once completed, you'll be able to see where you need to improve your skills and gain the confidence to successfully manage your own healthcare! Be open and honest with yourself as you complete this assessment. You probably know a lot more about your own lysosomal storage disease than you think. We recommend taking this assessment every year, beginning at age 14. This will give you time to fill in the gaps that are age-specific and help break your learning curve up into smaller pieces. It will also allow you to compare your progress annually as you make the transition to owning and managing your own healthcare.

Ready to Manage Your Own Healthcare Assessment Tool[3]

Initials: Date: Grade:

Directions: Read the following statements in the left-hand column. Find an answer to the right of the question that best sounds like you. Select only one answer per question.

A. General Medical Information	Agree	Sort of Agree and/or I've done it before	Sort of Disagree	Disagree or haven't done this yet	Does not apply
1. I know about my medical insurance and I carry an insurance card.					
2. I take good care of myself.					
3. I know where my private medical records are kept.					
4. I know how to get my health questions answered.					
5. If there was a medical emergency, I know who to contact and where to go.					
6. I think smoking, drinking, and drugs affect my health.					
7. I find it easy to fall asleep at night.					
8. I see the value of yearly visits to a doctor.					
9. I know how to use transportation to get to medical appointments.					
10. I schedule my own doctor appointments.					
11. I have a doctor who takes care of adult patients, not just kids.					
12. I know all about my physical changes in becoming an adult (like puberty, sexuality, pregnancy and sexually transmitted diseases).					

3. Project Youth, 1999 by Pacer Center, Inc. pacer@pacer.org Modified for Lysosomal Storage Diseases

B. Personal and Professional Interactions	Agree	Sort of Agree and/or I've done it before	Sort of Disagree	Disagree or haven't done this yet	Does not apply
13. It is easy to talk to doctors about my health concerns and issues.					
14. I like to have someone with me when I visit my doctor.					
15. I have someone to talk to when I feel sad.					
16. If needed, I know who to call and when with regards to my healthcare.					
17. I am not embarrassed about my lysosomal storage disease.					

C. Disability or Health Condition	Agree	Sort of Agree and/or I've done it before	Sort of Disagree	Disagree or haven't done this yet	Does not apply
18. I know a lot about my lysosomal storage disease.					
19. I feel like I control my lysosomal storage disease, it doesn't control me.					
20. I do not worry about my health.					
21. I think my lysosomal storage disease is under control and will not get in the way of what I want to do in the future.					
22. I know how to get my own personal care assistant or nurse (if you have a disability).					

D. Medications & Treatments	Agree	Sort of Agree and/or I've done it before	Sort of Disagree	Disagree or haven't done this yet	Does not apply
23. I know how to get my medications and enzyme replacement therapy (ERT).					
24. I think my medications will make a difference in my life.					
25. I know how to get and refill prescriptions and over-the-counter medications.					
26. I know the names of the medications I take and when I need to take them.					
TOTAL: Add the total check marks in each column and record it to the right.					

Now that you have answered items 1-26, let's look at the column entitled "Sort of Disagree" and "Disagree." If you have any check marks in those columns, it's time to take a closer look at addressing these items. Look at the shaded categories (A-D) in which they are organized. Then, on the next page, find the section for each category and read the discussion.

A. General Medical Information

Your age will have a lot of bearing on how you answered the questions in this section. At 14 years of age, you may not understand insurance or carry a card in your wallet; however, by age 18, this should be fully understood. This section is a guide so that by 18 years of age, you should agree with all statements. If you are 18 years old and you feel like you don't agree with all the statements on this tool, please talk to your physician, parent(s) or case manager and let's get started in getting you up to speed!

B. Personal and Professional Interactions

Knowing where to turn when you have a question or concern is probably the most important part of all in becoming independent in your own healthcare! Having a good relationship with a healthcare professional is essential in this transition period. It is also OK to have a friend come with you to the doctor so you have two sets of ears instead of one. There is data to suggest that when we visit the doctor with a specific problem, it is often the 5th concern we share! If you have a limited amount of time, you may not ever get to talk about the real reason for your visit. Don't be embarrassed or afraid to ask a question. Your doctor has heard it all! If you feel sad or depressed, let your doctor know. Many of the patient support groups, such as the National Fabry Disease Foundation (NFDF) have mentor and mental health programs that can help you through this transition period.

C Disability or Health Condition

Knowledge is power. Understanding your lysosomal storage disease is important to taking control of your health. It's the difference in knowing when to call the doctor or call the hospital. At 14 years of age, you should have a fundamental working knowledge of your disease and the primary parts of your body that are affected. You should know if your condition has more than one name such as "Hunter Syndrome", "Mucopolysaccharidosis Type II", and "MPSII" or "Pompe Disease" and "acid maltase deficiency." It is also important to know if you are you in the best health possible. If you have a disability due to your disease, do you have a personal care assistant or nurse to help with activities of daily living? There are abundant resources to help you live with a lysosomal storage disease, from patient support organizations to speaking with a genetic counselor and/or patient care liaison. These resources are listed in the back of this module.

D. Medications & Treatments

Just as understanding your disease is important, understanding the treatment and medication you are taking is also important.

You may discover that you are your nurse's only patient with Fabry disease or Hunter disease and their experience may be limited. Did you know that you probably couldn't walk up to your local pharmacy and order ERT? It either will come directly from the manufacturer or from a specialty pharmacy. Did you know that due to the fact that ERT is a protein, special mixing instructions need followed; you should never shake the protein or freeze the vials. It is important that you follow the directions of your physician and understand all your over-the-counter medications. Always ask a physician before taking an over-the-counter medication. Not all ERT has the same schedule; some are given weekly, while some are administered every other week. If you plan on missing an infusion, discuss making up the dose with your nurse or physician. Typically, you will want to space the make-up infusion about 3 to 7 days apart from your last infusion or next infusion. If you know a holiday is approaching, it is really important that you think ahead and determine when is the best time to make up your infusion.

Because many of the generic names for the enzymes sound alike, it is vitally important that you take an active role in knowing the names of your own medications. You will find a chart on the next page that may help. You can also share it with your nurse and/or doctor. Please correct healthcare professionals if they used the wrong name of your medication. Incorrect documentation of your disease or drug name can lead to medical errors.

Joining Research Projects

The decision to join a research study or experiment should be thought about carefully. Is the study just tracking the assessments you do (like a registry) or are they learning more about a possible new treatment? The doctors and coordinators running the studies will explain this to you using an informed consent as a guide. Don't be afraid to ask questions! Do not be afraid to say no, not every study is a good match for every person. No one will be mad or upset with you if you don't join a study.

Interested in Research?

Ask your LSD treatment team if anything is available for you. The support groups are also a good place to look for studies in your area. Additionally, all studies now register on www.ClinicalTrials.gov, a registry of federally and privately supported clinical trials conducted in the United States and around the world. ClinicalTrials.gov gives you information about a research trial's purpose, who may participate, locations, and phone numbers for more details. This information should be used in conjunction with advice from your medical team.

Some Common Medications Listed by Disease

Trade Name	Generic Name	Route of Administration	Manufacturer	Mechanism of Action	FDA Status
Cystinosis					
Cystagon™	cysteamine bitartrate	Oral	Mylan Pharmaceuticals Inc	cystine-depleting agent	Approved 1994
Procysbi™	cysteamine bitartrate, delayed release	Oral	Raptor Pharmaceuticals	cystine-depleting agent	Approved 2013
Cystaran™	Cysteamine hydrochloride	Eye drops	Sigma-Tau Pharmaceuticals, Inc	cystine-depleting agent	Approved 2012
Fabry Disease					
Fabrazyme™	Agalsidase beta	IV	Genzyme	ERT	Approved 2003
Replagal™	Agalsidase alfa	IV	Shire	ERT	Not approved in United States, but available in Europe/Canada
Not yet determined	AT1001	Oral	Amicus	Chaperone	Phase III clinical trials (2013)
Not yet determined	plant cell expressed recombinant human alpha-galactosidase-A (PRX-102)	IV	Protalix	ERT	Phase I/II clinical trials
Gaucher Disease					
Cerezyme™	Imiglucerase (injection)	IV	Genzyme	ERT	Approved 1994
VPRIV™	Velaglucerase alfa (injection)	IV	Shire	ERT	Approved 2010
Ceredase™	Alglucerase (injection)	IV	Genzyme	ERT	Approved 1991
Zavesca™	Miglustat	Oral	Actelion	SRT	Approved 2004
Elelyso™	Taliglucerase alfa	IV	Pfizer /Protalix	ERT	Approved 2012
Not yet determined	Eliglustat tartrate Genz-112638	Oral	Genzyme	SRT	Phase III Clinical Trial (2013)
Hurler/Hurler Scheie/Scheie (MPS I)					
Aldurazyme™	Laronidase	IV	Genzyme	ERT	Approved 2003
Hunter Disease (MPS II)					
Elaprase™	Idursulfase	IV	Shire	ERT	Approved 2006
Lysosomal Acid Lipase (LAL) Deficiency					
Not yet determined	sebelipase alfa (SBC-102	IV	Synageva		Phase III (2013)
Morquio (MPS IVA)					
Not yet determined	N-acetylgalactosa mine-6-sulfatase (BMN 110)	IV	BioMarin	ERT	Phase III Clinical Trial (2013)
Marateaux-Lamy (MPS VI)					
Naglazyme™	Galsulfase	IV	BioMarin	ERT	Approved 2005
Niemann-Pick Type C					
Zavesca™	Miglustat	Oral	Actelion	SRT	Off-label use only U.S.
Pompe Disease					
Myozyme™	Alglucosidase alfa	IV	Genzyme	ERT	Approved 2006
Lumizyme™	Alglucosidase alfa	IV	Genzyme	ERT	Approved for adults 2011

What are Chaperone, SRT, and ERT?

Chaperone therapy – A treatment that uses small molecules, usually taken as a pill, to help the body's own enzymes work better to clear away the stored material.

Enzyme replacement therapy (ERT) – IV infusion treatments which provide or "replace" an enzyme in individuals affected by an enzyme deficiency.

Substrate reduction therapy (SRT) – A treatment (usually in pill form) which reduces the amount of material that an enzyme needs to break down by preventing the stored material from being created in the first place.

Chapter Six
Autonomy Checklist for Adolescents

(modified from checklist developed by the Youth in Transition Project (1984-1987) University of Washington Division of Adolescent Medicine and based on a model developed by the Children's Rehabilitation Center at the University of Virginia.)

Autonomy: noun; independence or freedom, as of the will or one's actions: the autonomy of the individual

Step 1: Skills **Instructions:** To the right of each item, check the box that best describes you.	I Do This Already	I Probably Need a Little Help or Practice	I Plan to Start Working on This
Understand my health status			
Am aware of existence of medical records, diagnosis information, etc.			
Prepare questions for my doctors, nurses, therapists			
Respond to questions from my doctors, nurses, therapists			
Know my medications and what they treat			
Can get a prescription filled			
Know the dose of treatment and how often I receive it			
Understand the side effects that could occur with my medications			
Manage my insurance issues			
Keep a calendar of doctor, dentist, and other healthcare appointments			
Know my height, weight, and birth date			
Know how to read a thermometer			
Know health emergency telephone numbers			
Know medical coverage numbers such as Social Security number or group policy numbers			
Obtain sex education materials/birth control as needed			
Know what my treatment and assessment plan is and where to find it			
Have had genetic counseling about my condition and its inheritance in my family			
Discuss drugs and alcohol with my family			
Make contact with appropriate community advocacy organization (i.e. FSIG, NGF)			
(If female) Take care of own menstrual needs and keep a record of monthly periods			
Can get to my own appointments, know directions			

Step 1: Skills (continued)	I Do This Already	I Probably Need a Little Help or Practice	I Plan to Start Working on This
Understand what it means to live on my own			
Have a good understanding of budgets and financial considerations			
Know what my educational plans are after high school			
Fill out job employment applications on-line or hard-copy applications by myself			
Fill out insurance forms on my own			

Step 2: Score

Instructions: Tally how many check marks you have in the PLAN TO START column in Step 1. Record that number in the box to the right.

Step 3: Action Plan

Instructions: Take a close look at all the items that you have checked in the Plan to Start column (in Step 1). Choose 3 of them (if you have 3 or more) and write them below. Together, with your family or support team, identify a responsible person to help you complete the action. It might be that more than one person is responsible for the action. If you would like to accept responsibility to learn and grow, now is your time!

In the right-hand column, place the date you wish to accomplish the action item. It is important to also ask the question, *"How will I know I've mastered the action?"* Some actions will be obvious; for instance, "Make my own doctor's appointment." Of course, you would know if that was completed. However, what if one of the action items is to "Understand your disease better." How will you know you have mastered this? As you go through this exercise with your family, listening to each other and to members of your support team is a critical step. Remember, our fears are strong motivators of our behavior.

Issue/Need/or Concern Identified	Who will help you with this task?	How will you know when you master this task?	Date you would like to complete task
Example: I don't know how to order my enzyme replacement therapy in college	My case manager	There is a shipment date for your medication.	Before August 15
1.			
2.			
3.			

Chapter Seven
Transition Planning to Manage your Healthcare

Think back to one of your favorite vacations. As young children, we packed our favorite stuffed animal in our suitcase, maybe our toothbrush, and away we went. Not much planning on our part, was there? As young adults, we may have been asked where we wanted to go on vacation and the next thing we knew we were on our way. Did that vacation just happen or was actual planning involved? Well, like vacation planning, transition planning is an integral part of our success in managing our own healthcare as young adults.

What is a Transition Plan?

A transition plan is typically a **written plan** based on the needs and issues that should be addressed prior to a teen transitioning to adult care. Many people should have input into this plan, but especially you! As the one doing the transitioning, you may have concerns, issues, and needs that need to be taken into account! It's important this plan be tailored to YOU specifically, as no two people are alike.

Identifying the transition needs and issues is the first step. Once these needs/issues/concerns have been outlined, action steps should be developed to address each issue. Each **action step** should have a responsible person and a date by which the action should be completed. If you feel you are ready and responsible to accept an action item, it might take a little convincing with the adults in your life. One of the hardest parts for your parents and/or guardian is realizing you aren't a kid any longer and that you are growing up. It is important to remember that these action steps will need continual updating and that you can add to the list at any point. The goal is to get you to think ahead, anticipate future needs, and be able to problem solve on your own, or by obtaining the help of others. Start with the forms we have provided at the end of this module. Modify them or find better ones if you'd like. It's your transition, after all! Additionally, knowing your resources is half the battle. We have added resources at the end of this module for you to use.

Chapter Eight
Knowing your Resources

Remember, you are not alone just because you are on your own and/or transitioning to independence. Many resources are available to you. For example, if you work, your Human Resources (HR) Department can help answer many questions about insurance or benefits with your new job. The medical clinic at many universities can help with infusion questions and your local physician may be able to help you identify a primary care physician in your new city or town. And finally, your local doctor, genetic counselor, and your parents, are often only a phone call away!

Overall Resources:

A detailed booklet on *"Adolescent transition care: A Guidance for nursing staff"* http://www.rcn.org.uk/__data/assets/pdf_file/0011/78617/002313.pdf

Health Knowledge Questionnaire *"Ready to Manage Your Own Health Care?"* http://www.minnesotaschoolnurses.org/Ready_to_Manage_Questionnaire.pdf

Several useful Transition Questionnaires and Resources can be found at http://www.minnesotaschoolnurses.org/ in the special education section.

Disease and treatment summary sheets: several paper-based options at http://depts.washington.edu/healthtr/, as well as digital options, such as the iPHONE application called **My Med ID**

Additional parent and Teen-focused transition worksheets and resources in English and Spanish: http://internet.dscc.uic.edu/dsccroot/parents/transition.asp

A really nice transition discussion: http://www.gottransition.org/

Detailed summaries about genetic conditions including the LSDs: http://www.ncbi.nlm.nih.gov/sites/GeneTests/review?db=genetests

More Resources!
(alphabetical by condition name)

Cystinosis Resources

There are multiple support options for patients with cystinosis.

The Cystinosis Foundation is a non-profit organization with more than 25 years of international experience in supporting and educating families and the medical community through the dissemination of educational literature, funding research, and annual conferences. http://www.cystinosisfoundation.org/

The Cystinosis Research Network is an all-volunteer, non-profit organization dedicated to supporting and advocating research, providing family assistance and educating the public and medical communities about Cystinosis. https://cystinosis.org

The Cystinosis Research Foundation's mission is two-fold and focused: to find better treatments and a cure for cystinosis. Funding quality research studies remains a priority and is an ongoing process. http://www.natalieswish.com

Information on treatment with Cystagon capsules from CVS CAREMARK Pharmacy, in partnership with Mylan Pharmaceutical, can be obtained by calling 1-800-238-7828

Information about the Procysbi treatment for Cystinosis by the manufacturer (Raptor) can be found at: http://www.procysbi.com/

More information about eye specific treatment for cystinosis can be found at the pharmaceutical website: http://www.cystaran.com/

Fabry Disease Resources

Resources and support for Fabry disease are numerous. The National Fabry Disease Foundation (NFDF) (www.fabrydisease.org/) and Fabry Support and Information Group (FSIG) (www.fabry.org) are United States support groups available to provide information about Fabry disease. The organizations also set up group meetings and offer insurance support. Membership is free to both organizations. Information about upcoming clinical research trials is also available on their websites and can help you stay current in regard to clinical research. You may enjoy the message boards that are offered, as well as webcasts that relay important information. These groups also have active Facebook pages you can join.

Many pharmaceutical companies offer case management support and help navigating insurance issues. These services are free. Case managers can help you with prior authorization for ERT, verify insurance, and help answer questions you have about your insurance benefits. If you are interested in this service talk to your healthcare provider or access the company's website.

For additional Fabry information that is easy to comprehend and understand, visit www.fabrycommunity.com. For treatment information, visit www.fabrazyme.com. Information can be easily downloaded for educational purposes.

Clinical trial information regarding other upcoming therapies can be found at **www.clinicaltrials.gov**.

Gaucher Disease Resources

Since the arrival of newer therapy options on the market for those living with Gaucher disease, new resources for people living with Gaucher disease have also arrived. With well over 1500 patients receiving ERT for Gaucher disease every year in the United States, you are not alone!

The National Gaucher Foundation (NGF)
The National Gaucher Foundation (NGF), a non-profit organization established in 1984, has donated millions of dollars to support and promote research towards the cause, treatments and a cure for Gaucher disease. To meet the ever-increasing needs of individuals with Gaucher disease and their families, The NGF offers a wide range of programs and resources for the benefit of the Gaucher community. The NGF sponsors research, offers financial assistance, promotes education and awareness, supports legislative issues and provides outreach programs vital to the Gaucher community. Through The National Gaucher Care Foundation, the CARE Program and the Care+Plus Program provide critical financial assistance to individuals with Gaucher Disease. In support of medical and lay community awareness, the NGF holds live Web meetings, national conferences, patient meetings and seminars, and runs national and regional marketing programs.

You can find the NGF at www.gaucherdisease.org, or by calling toll-free 1-800-504-3189.

Shire offers their OnePathSM Services, a billing and resources support system for patients, families and healthcare

providers. This is a free service that provides assistance with reimbursement and insurance verification. OnePath Services offers a dedicated case manager Monday-Friday, 8:30 am to 8:00 pm EST. They can be reached at 1-866-888-0660, or on the web at www.onepath.com.

Genzyme Treatment Support also provides comprehensive services to those living with Gaucher disease. Specialized case managers will help you navigate through important insurance considerations and help answer questions related to insurance, co-pays, and verification. They can be reached toll-free at 800-745-4447 or 617-768-9000. You can visit them online at www.genzyme.com.

Pfizer offers Gaucher Personal Support , a billing and resources support system for patients, families and healthcare providers. This is a free service that provides assistance with reimbursement and insurance verification. They can be reached 24 hours a day at 1-855-ELELYSO (1-855-353-5976) or online at http://www.elelyso.com/gps.aspx .

Disease and treatment-specific information can also be found at:

www.gauchercare.com
www.ngf.org
www.cerezyme.com
www.bravecommunity.com
www.gaucherpatients.com
www.shire.com
www.vpriv.com
www.protalix.com/Patients/ProtalixPatientsCare.html

Krabbe

The primary support resource for Krabbe Disease (also known as Globoid Cell Leukodystrophy) is the advocacy and support group Hunter's Hope Foundation (http://www.huntershope. org) Additional resources and information about clinical trials/treatment for Krabbe Disease can be found at The United Leukodystrophy Foundation (www.ulf.org).

LAL Deficiency Resources

The primary support resource for Lysosomal Acid Lipase Deficiency (LAL Deficiency also known as Cholesteryl ester storage disease) is the support group LAL Solace found at http://www.lalsolace.org/ . Additional resources and information about clinical trials/treatment for LAL deficiency can be found at Synageva BioPharma Corporation's informational website: http://www.laldeficiencysource.com/

Mucolipidosis Types II & III/ Glycoprotein Disorders Resources

The principle resources and support for ML II/III and other glycoprotein conditions can be found through the ISMRD. The ISMRD is an internationally focused nonprofit organization whose mission is to advocate for families and patients affected by one of the Glycoprotein Storage Diseases. Their website can be found at: www.ismrd.org

MPS Resources

The National MPS Society exists to support and find cures for MPS and related diseases. They provide hope and support for people living with the disease and their families, through research, advocacy and awareness of these devastating diseases. Locate the National MPS Society on the web at www.mpssociety.org or by calling toll-free 1-877-MPS-1001.

The National Organization for Rare Disorders (NORD) can be found at www.rarediseases.org. While this organization is not specific for MPS, they do offer patient assistance programs, insight into clinical research and support for patients and families.

And lastly, a parent and/or young adult message board can be found at www.MPSforum.com

MPS I Disease (Hurler, Hurler Scheie and/or Scheie) Resources

MPS I disease has a wide disease spectrum, ranging from a mild form to a more severe form. Support for individuals and families is mainly available through the National MPS Society at www.mpssociety.org. Many of the patient and family meetings will encompass all of the MPS diseases, so you'll find patients with Hurler syndrome as well as other MPS syndromes. Other information is available through Genzyme at http://www.mps1disease.com.

Can you explain the links between BioMarin, Genzyme, and Aldurazyme?

BioMarin manufactures the enzyme replacement therapy medication for MPSI, called Aldurazyme. Genzyme promotes and sells Aldurazyme. Genzyme will help you understand your insurance policy, your co-pays, and help you find an infusion center. You can reach Genzyme by calling toll-free 1-800-745-4447 or going to www.genzyme.com.

Disease-specific information can be found at www.MPSIdisease.com and drug information can be accessed at www.aldurazyme.com.

Parent and Teen message board can also be accessed at http://www.mpsforum.com

MPSII (Hunter Disease) Resources

In addition to the overall MPS resources, such as the National MPS Society (www.mpssociety.org), people with MPSII or Hunter disease also have some more specific support resources to help in their transition to adulthood and managing their own healthcare.

The Hunter Patient site, http://www.hunterpatients.com, is a patient-friendly site that keeps families updated and informed.

From the billing and insurance perspective, the maker of Elaprase, Shire HGT, provides a free service called OnePathSM Services. This support service provides you with a dedicated case manager to help answer your questions about reimbursement, insurance verification, help in locating an infusion center and much more. You can reach them toll-free at 1-866-888-0660 or on the web at: www.onepath.com.

MPSIII (Sanfilippo syndrome) Resources

The National MPS Society provides several important support resources and updates on clinical research studies for individuals with MPSIII. The National MPS Society website can be found at: www.mpssociety.org

MPSIV (Morquio syndrome) Resources

In addition to the overall MPS resources, such as the National MPS Society (www.mpssociety.org), there are also support resources such as the Carol Ann Foundation at http://www.morquio.com/ . The Carol Ann Foundation holds annual meetings about MPSIV and works closely with researchers studying the condition. More information about the research and progress on enzyme replacement therapy for MPSIV can be found on the BioMarin website at http://www.biomarinclinicaltrials.com/MPSIVA.html

MPS VI Disease (Maroteaux-Lamy) Resources

BioMarin manufactures, promotes and distributes the drug Naglazyme for the treatment of Maroteaux-Lamy disease. Most of the patient and family support can be gleaned from attending a meeting hosted by the MPS Society. For more information on meetings close to you, please visit www.mpssociety.org.

For patient advocacy, visit www.biomarin.com or www.bmrn.com. BioMarin Patient and Physicians Support (BPPS) can also be found here.

A parent message board can be accessed at http://www.mpsforum.com.

The National Organization for Rare Disorders (NORD) is dedicated to helping people with rare, orphan diseases. While not specific to MPS VI disease, information, support and special events can be found at: www.raredisease.org.

Niemann Pick Resources

There are 3 very different types of health condition (A, B, and C) all called Niemann Pick. The National Niemann-Pick Disease Foundation (http://www.nnpdf.org/) provides information and support for all 3 NP types. Specific Information about Niemann-Pick type C can also be found at the Ara Parseghian Medical Research Foundation at http://www.parseghian.org/

Pompe Disease Resources

Resources and Support for Pompe Disease range from patient support groups to pharmaceutical company resources focused on treatment. The primary Pompe support links are listed below:

Acid Maltase Deficiency Association (AMDA)-- Phone: (210) 494-6144 or (210) 490-7161 www.amda-pompe.org

Association for Glycogen Storage Disease http://www.agsdus.org/

United Pompe Foundation http://www.unitedpompe.com

Muscular Dystrophy Association (MDA http://www.mdausa.org/

National Organization for Rare Disorders, Inc. (NORD) http://www.rarediseases.org/

Clinical Trials.gov--Information on research for Pompe disease can be found at: http://clinicaltrials.gov/search/term=Pompe%20Disease Office of Rare Diseases http://rarediseases.info.nih.gov

Pompe Community (information provided by Genzyme Therapeutics) http://www.pompe.com/patient/pc_eng_pt_main.asp

In addition, specific information regarding treatment and enzyme replacement therapy can be found at www.myozyme.com. Genzyme, the manufacturer of Myozyme and Lumizyme, sponsors this site.

Late Onset Tay-Sachs Resources

The primary support resources for Late Onset Tay Sachs is the Late Onset Tay-Sachs Research and Education Foundation. (http://www.lateonsettay-sachs.org/)

The Foundation was established in 2007 to educate and help people affected with this debilitating disease that strikes older children, teens and adults alike.

Chapter Nine

Your Own Plan

Name: _____ Date: _____

DOB: _____

Disease: _____

ICD9 Code*: _____

People identified to help me complete my transition plan:

1. _____
2. _____
3. _____

Doctors I need to see, their specialty and the reason I need to see them:

1. _____ Specialty: _____

   Reason: _____ Appt. Date: _____

2. _____ Specialty: _____

   Reason: _____ Appt. Date: _____

3. _____ Specialty: _____

   Reason: _____ Appt. Date: _____

4. _____ Specialty: _____

   Reason: _____ Appt. Date: _____

5. _____ Specialty: _____

   Reason: _____ Appt. Date: _____

6. _____ Specialty: _____

   Reason: _____ Appt. Date: _____

*ICD9 Codes are the numbers used to identify and classify specific health conditions. Some examples are: Gaucher & Fabry Disease: 272.7 MPS conditions: 277.5 Pompe Disease: 271.0

My Treatment Plan

I have obtained a **Schedule of Assessments** for my disease: ☐ Yes ☐ No

If NO is checked, what plan do you have to obtain this valuable tool? There is no charge for this tool. It is available via the web in most instances. Sharing this with your healthcare team will help you get the best care possible!

Medications:

Name of Medication: _____

☐ ERT ☐ SRT ☐ Other _____

Pre-medications (i.e. medication to take before ERT): ☐ Yes ☐ No

    If yes, please list here: _____

_____

Dose of Medication (i.e. how much): _____

Frequency (i.e. how often): _____

Duration (i.e. how long) as applicable: _____

Rate (as applicable): ☐ Yes ☐ No

Side effects to watch for during an infusion: _____

_____

Have you had an infusion reaction in the past?: ☐ Yes ☐ No

    If yes, please describe: _____

_____

Other medications (list name, dose, reason taking, prescription, over-the-counter, what side effect(s) you've had): _____

_____

_____

Health symptoms that should be on my radar screen:

1. _____

2. _____

3. _____

How will you get to and from your appointments?

_____

Health History Forms

Health History or Medical History forms are very, very useful in understanding your LSD condition, your health, and your treatment. Completing a version of this form with your parent(s) or health care provider creates an easily found place to jog your memory and introduce yourself to new physicians. Keeping this tool updated as new things occur is important.

There are several good ways to track this information, ranging from paper forms to iPhones apps. Please see some options below:

Adolescent Health Transition Project: Health History Summary form is available in several languages including: English, Chinese, Korean, Russian, Spanish, and Vietnamese:
http://depts.washington.edu/healthtr/resources/tools/forms.html

iPhone Apps:
My Med ID
My Medical, by Hyrax Inc.
OnePath Gaucher (for Gaucher disease)

Android Apps:
My Medical Info
My Health Records - Health n Family
ICE: In Case of Emergency, by Appventive

Medical information jewelry
Medic Alert Foundation http://www.medicalert.org/
Sticky Jewelry http://www.stickyj.com/
Medical USB http://www.medictag.com/

Example letter that you may wish to use to introduce yourself to your new doctors when you schedule your first appointment:

Your Name

Your Address

Your Doctor's Name

Your Doctor's Address

Date:

Dear Doctor _____,

I am writing this letter to tell you a little bit about myself and my genetic condition. This letter is part of my transition plan to take charge of my medical care now that I am an adult.

I am affected by a genetic condition called _____. This disease is a progressive lysosomal storage disease that affects most of the organs in my body. I have attached a great review summary of my condition for your review, my treatment plan, and my personal medical history summary sheet. As you can see, it is very important that I work closely with my doctors to manage my condition's symptoms. Previously, my parents and my pediatric specialists have helped me to make doctors appointments and make medical decisions. Although my parents will still help me, I am transitioning to adult doctors and may need some extra time with you as I learn the adult medicine system. Please be patient with me.

In addition to my visits with you, I will be continuing to see my genetics team as well as other physicians. My genetics team can be reached at _____. Prior to my appointments, I will try and let your office know about any hospitalizations, surgeries, or other medical appointments, so that you can gather and review records as needed before my appointments. Please let me know the best way to contact your office to make appointments and know any other appointments with other doctors.

I am excited and a little anxious to be moving forward into adulthood. Thank you for being part of my journey.

Sincerely,

Your Name

Enclosure: Personal medical history summary and GeneClinics review article

For Your Parents

Suggestions for your parents as they help young adults transition to managing their healthcare

- Talk with your teen about their healthcare. Learn what he or she thinks about managing his or her own care.

- Identify the healthcare skills that your teen can already perform, the skills he or she needs to learn, and the skills requiring help. For example, some teens may not be able to talk about the medications they take, but can carry information in their wallets or phones.

- Teach your teen any danger signs associated with his or her condition. Develop a plan of action for your teen to follow when the danger signs are present.

- Encourage your teen to schedule and prepare for his or her own medical appointments.

- Encourage your teen to talk to his or her doctor (and other healthcare providers) and to ask questions.

- Identify people who can address health issues in planning the transition for your teen. It may be a physician, school nurse, teacher, or family member. Goals for learning about one's disorder or disability are appropriate for the IEP.

- Consider choosing a physician who can take over the healthcare of your teen once he or she is an adult. Meet with the doctor, so he or she is familiar with your teen's needs.

- Identify a health advocate, if needed. It can be a family member or a friend who will interact with healthcare providers on behalf of your teen if he or she needs assistance or is unable to communicate clearly for him or herself.

- Teach your teen (at all ages) basic life skills, providing ample opportunity to practice problem-solving and management skills. Identify areas that require extra attention.

- Discuss career goals with your teen.

- Take good care of yourself — parents and other family members are role models for children and teens of all ages!!!

Brief Transitions Glossary

Case manager – A healthcare professional assigned to assist individuals and families cope with complicated health or medical situations in the most effective way possible. This often includes help with planning, coordination, monitoring, and evaluation of medical services for a patient, with emphasis on quality of care, continuity of services, and cost-effectiveness

Chaperone therapy – A treatment that uses small molecules, usually taken as a pill, to help the body's own enzymes work better to reduce the stored material.

Clinical summary – A document that lists your important medical information, both past and present

Clinical trial – A medical research study investigating specific medical questions in humans. Many studies are focused on the safety and effectiveness of new medications. In the United States, many clinical trials are rigorously controlled and conducted under the supervision of the Food and Drug Administration (FDA).

Co-pay – short for co-payment, this is a small fixed amount of money that your health insurance company requires you contribute in paying for each medical visit or prescription

Cystinosis – A genetic condition which causes a substance called cysteine to build up within the body's cells and form crystals which can damage the body's organs, particularly the kidneys and the eyes.

Deductible – A specific amount of money that you must pay before your insurance company will begin to pay for your treatment.

Enzyme – A chemical or protein which causes or speeds up biochemical reactions in the body (such as the digestion of food or the breakdown of stored up material). In lysosomal storage diseases, the body does not make enough of a particular enzyme and/or the enzyme is not working properly and cannot breakdown stored up material.

Enzyme replacement therapy (ERT) – IV infusion treatments which provide or "replace" an enzyme in individuals affected by an enzyme deficiency.

Explanation of Benefits (EOB) – A form that may be sent to you by your health insurance company several months after you receive medical care, explaining which parts of the medical care were paid by the insurance company on your behalf.

Fabry – A genetic condition in which an enzyme called "alpha-galactosidase A" (a-gal A) is not being produced by the body in sufficient amounts, causing a substance called "globotriaosylceramide" (GL3 or GB3) to build up within the body's cells and damage the body's organs, particularly the heart and the kidneys. Other symptoms often include pain in the hands and feet, fatigue, and an inability to sweat.

Gaucher – A genetic condition in which an enzyme called "beta-glucocerebrosidase" is not being produced by the body in sufficient amounts, causing a substance called "glucocerebroside" to build up within the body's cells and cause disease symptoms including: low blood iron and platelets, fatigue, and an enlarged liver and spleen. Other symptoms often include bone pain and poor growth.

Genetics – A branch of biology that studies how personal and medical traits, characteristics, and diseases are inherited or "passed down" in families.

Genetic Counselor – A person with expertise in genetics who helps individuals and families determine if they have or are at risk for a genetic disorder, as well as giving them information about the disorder, including the risk of passing it on to their children. The counselor can explain the medical science involved, help identify available treatment options, and provide general support.

Geneticist – A doctor who specializes in medical diseases and conditions that are inherited or "passed down" in families.

Health insurance – An agreement with a company that in return for your (or your employer's) paying them a regular amount every month, they will pay for most of your medical and surgical expenses if you get sick (See chapter 3 for more details about different kinds of health insurance).

Health Insurance Portability and Accountability Act (HIPAA) – A federal act in 1995 which established national standards to protect an individual's medical records and other personal health information (which is sometimes referred to as PHI).

In-network doctor – A doctor who is contracted with your insurance company, which means you pay less money for your doctor visits, tests, etc.

Individualized Education Program (IEP) – Created by the Individuals with Disabilities Education Act, this is a service allowing children and teens with delayed skills or other disabilities to have the services and programs they need to help them succeed in the public school system. Parents of children with special needs work together with educators to develop a personal plan to help their child. At 16 years of age, a teenager has the right to be a part of their IEP transition team. This service is free of charge.

Infusion – A medical procedure that injects liquid medication into the body using a needle and a small tube, temporarily inserted into a vein, often in a person's arm.

Intravenous (IV) therapy – giving medication by infusion

Lipid – a fat molecule in the body which is not water-soluble (i.e. does not dissolve in water)

Lysosomal storage diseases (LSD) – A set of diseases in which a particular enzyme needed by the body to break down extra material is not present or is not being made in great enough quantities. As a result, the unwanted material begins to collect and be "stored" in the cells of the body in the lysosome, causing various physical symptoms, depending on the disease.

Lysosome – The cell's recycling and disposal center. They are located in every cell in the body and contain enzymes that digest the unwanted material.

Mucopolysaccharidosis (MPS) – A group of genetic conditions in which one or more enzymes needed to break down substances called "glycosaminoglycans" or "GAGs" are not being produced by the body in sufficient amount, causing GAGs to build up within the body's cells and damage the body's organs and/or bones.

Out-of- network doctor – A doctor who may accept your insurance, but does not work as closely with your insurance company. This may mean that you are responsible for paying a higher portion of your medical bill.

Peripheral access – The placement of a small flexible tube into a vein in the body, usually on the hand or arm, in order to administer medication or fluids.

Pharmaceutical – related to medical drugs or a pharmacy

Pompe – A genetic condition in which an enzyme called "alpha-glucosidase" is not being produced by the body in sufficient amounts, causing a substance called "glycogen" to build up within the body's cells and damage the body's organs and tissues, particularly the muscles.

Port-a-cath (port) – A device placed under the skin, usually in the upper chest, to make it easier to access a person's veins, for people who need frequent infusions.

Pre-existing condition – A health problem that already exists before you apply for a health insurance policy or enroll in a new health plan.

Primary care physician (PCP) – A doctor who provides generalized care for medical problems, chosen by a person to serve as his or her main doctor and to coordinate their medical care as they need it, including making referrals to doctors who specialize in certain parts of the body when necessary.

Registry – An organized collection of data about a specific disease, so that doctors and researchers can use the data to learn more about the disease.

Specialty care physician – a doctor who specializes in a particular body system or branch of medicine, like the heart, lungs, or like genetics

Supplemental Security Income (SSI) – A United States government program that provides financial help to low-income people who are either older (65 years and up), blind, or disabled from working in some way.

Substrate – A substance in the body that an enzyme is trying to digest, break down, and recycle.

Substrate reduction therapy (SRT) – A treatment (usually in pill form) which reduces the amount of material that an enzyme needs to break down by preventing the stored material from being created.

References

Grinzaid, K, et al. Cessation of enzyme replacement therapy in Gaucher disease, *Genetics in Medicine*, November/December 2002, Vol. 4, No. 6.

iVillage.com, http://yourtotalhealth.ivallage.com/when-call-doctor.html, accessed 2012.

Project Youth, "Ready to Manage Your Own Health Care?" Pacer Center Inc., 1999. http://www.minnesotaschoolnurses.org.

Youth in Transition, "Autonomy Checklist for Adolescents" University of Washington Division of Adolescent Medicine. (1984-1987)

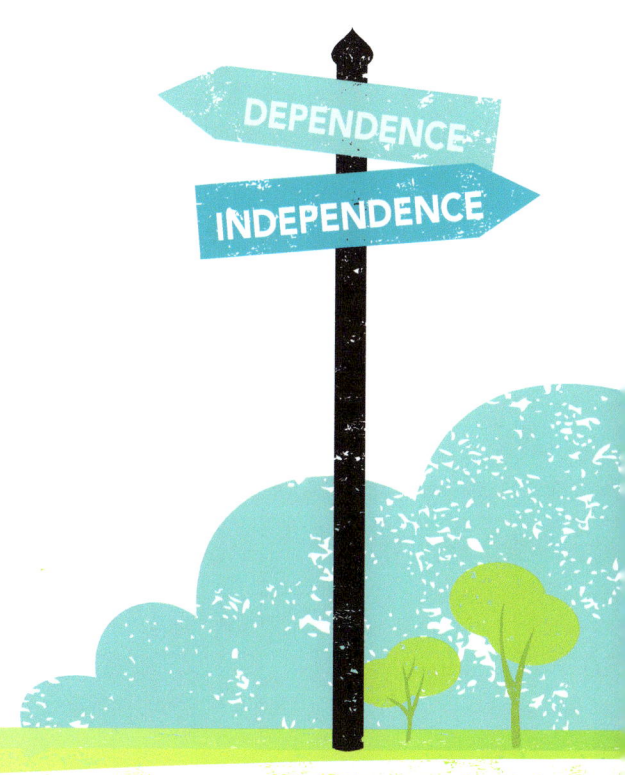